CHATGPT, MD

CHATGPT, MD

HOW AI-EMPOWERED PATIENTS & DOCTORS CAN TAKE BACK CONTROL OF AMERICAN MEDICINE

ROBERT PEARL, MD
& CHATGPT

This work incorporates text generated by artificial intelligence under the guidance and direction of Robert Pearl, MD. In accordance with the U.S. Copyright Office's requirements, the copyright claim for this work applies solely to the original content authored by Robert Pearl, MD, and does not extend to any material generated by AI. The use of AI-generated text is intended to enhance the reader's experience and provide additional insights, and is clearly indicated throughout the work. The copyright of this book protects only the human-authored content, and any use, reproduction, or distribution of the work must respect these boundaries.

Copyright © 2024 by Robert Pearl, assisted by ChatGPT
Cover design by Jonathan Pliego, assisted by Midjourney
Print book interior design by Clayton Smith, assisted by Adobe

All rights reserved. No part of this book may be scanned, uploaded, used, reproduced, or distributed in any manner whatsoever without written permission. If you would like permission to use material from the book (other than in the case of brief quotations embodied in articles and reviews), please contact lincolnliterary@outlook.com. Thank you for your support of authors' rights.

Printed in the United States of America
First Edition: April 2024
Published by Robert Pearl, MD

Library of Congress Control Number: 2024906826

Dr. Robert Pearl is available for media interviews and public-speaking events. To find out more visit his website www.robertpearlmd.com or email his publicist: Ben Lincoln at lincolnliterary@outlook.com.

Includes bibliographical references.
ISBN: 979-8-9903346-0-1 (hardcover), 979-8-9903346-1-8 (e-book)

For Janet, who shares my heart and my passion for healing.

CONTENTS

PART ONE: GENERATIONS

Chapter One	The Evolution of Medical Miracles	2
Chapter Two	ChatGPT and the Next Frontier	7
Chapter Three	The Life and Times of American Medicine	18
Chapter Four	Healthcare's Unfulfilled Promises	23
Chapter Five	Knowledge Is Power	34
Chapter Six	The AI Revolution: In ChatGPT's Own Words	39

PART TWO: GENERATIVITY

Chapter Seven	Welcome to Healthcare 4.0	46
Chapter Eight	A First Look at AI Empowerment	53
Chapter Nine	Fixing Medicine's Biggest Problems	60
Chapter Ten	The Doctor-Patient-AI Partnership	72

PART THREE: GENESIS

Chapter Eleven	The Road to AI-Empowered Healthcare	79
Chapter Eleven.five	ChatGPT's Critical Analysis of 'The Road to AI-Empowered Healthcare'	92
Chapter Twelve	Systemness	96
Chapter Thirteen	From Catalog Kings to Healthcare Disruptors	107
Chapter Fourteen	Breaking The Rules	119

PART FOUR: GENTLY

Chapter Fifteen	Ethics, Privacy, and Trust	134
Chapter Sixteen	Misinformation and Medical Credibility	150
Chapter Seventeen	The Human Element	161

PART FIVE: NEXT GEN

Chapter Eighteen	Technology Alone Is not Enough	177
Chapter Nineteen	The Fourth Pillar	184
Chapter Twenty	Pole Position	192
Chapter Twenty-one	Leadership: From A to G	197
Chapter Twenty-two	Seizing Serendipity	211
	Acknowledgments	*221*
	Bibliography	*225*

PART ONE
GENERATIONS

PART ONE | CHAPTER ONE

THE EVOLUTION OF MEDICAL MIRACLES

Picture yourself standing in the halls of Groote Schuur Hospital in Cape Town, South Africa, on December 3, 1967. You can sense that the air is charged with anticipation, nerves, and the undeniable sense that an historic moment is unfolding.

You watch as a 53-year-old grocer named Louis Washkansky is wheeled into one of the operating rooms. He has diabetes and severe heart failure. Without immediate surgery, he doesn't have long to live.

Soon, his life and the life of another patient will intersect in unprecedented fashion.

In the other surgical suite, a 25-year-old bank clerk named Denise Darvall is also being prepped for surgery. Yesterday, the young clerk had been the picture of perfect health when fate dealt a devastating blow. She and her mother had been shopping downtown when the two stepped off the curb to cross a busy street and, *wham*, a fast-moving vehicle collided with the young Darvall, severely damaging her body and destroying her brain.

In the first operating room where Washkansky lies, a pioneering cardiac surgeon named Christian Bernard splits the grocer's sternum down the middle with a power saw. He then places the patient on a cardiopulmonary bypass—allowing for a bloodless field on which to perform a surgical procedure that has never been attempted before.

In the second operating room, surgeons remove the heart and kidneys of the brain-dead donor. As the young woman's kidneys are rushed to a distant OR, another physician carries her heart through the entryway of the first surgical suite to the table where Dr. Bernard now stands beside Washkansky's unconscious body.

And here, in Cape Town, a heart once beating in one human is transplanted into another, marking a leap in medical science so profound that it borders on the miraculous. This is not just surgery taking place. It is a moment that will redefine the boundaries of medicine, turning the seemingly impossible into reality.

***

When I finished medical school at Yale, I chose Stanford University for my residency. I did so for the opportunity to work with Dr. Norman Shumway, the medical center's chief of cardiac surgery. A year after the first human heart transplant took place in Cape Town, Dr. Shumway performed the first "successful" heart transplant in the United States. I qualify that word because the recipient, a 54-year-old steel worker, lived only 14 days after the operation (four days fewer than the patient in Cape Town).

Despite the initial travails of this risky surgical procedure, the following decade created a nationwide burst of enthusiasm for heart transplantation. Although I would eventually choose plastic and reconstructive surgery for my specialty—having fallen in love with the beauty of cleft lip repair on global surgical missions—I'll never forget my days in the OR at Stanford with Dr. Shumway, a brilliant technical surgeon and dedicated medical pioneer.

By the time I arrived at Stanford, he had persevered in making cardiac transplantation safer and more reliable. Despite intense controversy over the legal and economic issues surrounding the procedure, alongside difficult ethical questions about what constitutes "brain death" in potential donors, Dr. Shumway and his team never gave up. The team advanced the operative technique decade upon decade, paving the way for a procedure that is now standard.

Looking back, as I contemplate the magnitude of risks that both patients and surgeons were willing to accept in those early days of heart transplantation, I'm struck by the arc of modern medicine. In this profession, again and again, the unimaginable becomes possible and then routine. Research from the 1980s shows that only 30 percent of patients survived five years post-transplant. Today, the long-term survival rate exceeds 80 percent.

***

American medicine now finds itself on the precipice of another revolutionary moment. This one is not taking place in an operating room but instead within the digital domains of generative AI. Technology that once seemed the stuff of science fiction is becoming pervasive.

Initially received with awe and disbelief in November 2022 when OpenAI released its large language model, ChatGPT, this "miraculous" technology is already developing into an integral part of daily life.

Dozens of industries—from retail and finance to consulting and entertainment—are investing billions of dollars to harness the full potential of ChatGPT and other forms of generative AI. There are, as of this book's publication, more than 300 different categories of AI tools on the market: from simple text-to-text generators to something called "NeRFs," neural radiance fields, which can be used to generate 3D imagery based on 2D images. With AI, you can even clone your own voice and use it to record an audiobook. More categories and use cases are surfacing constantly.

History teaches that today's technological miracles will become tomorrow's mundanities. Just as heart transplants moved from groundbreaking to standard care, generative AI will—in time—transition from a wondrous novelty to a technology people rely on as comfortably as they do their smartphones and computers. And, one day, this radical technology will transform medical practice, as well.

If you haven't tried any of the generative AI platforms yet, I encourage you to do so at the conclusion of this chapter. You will quickly find yourself as rapt as I did in spring 2023 when I began typing questions into ChatGPT (located at chat.openai.com).

One of my earliest requests was a simple query. I typed the following prompt into the message bar and tapped the return key.

"What is a miracle?"

At first, GPT-4 (the upgraded, subscription version of ChatGPT that launched in March 2023) responded as I had expected, providing a religious definition.

"An extraordinary event that is seen as a sign of God's supernatural power." But at the end of the answer, it pointed out, "The definition and interpretation of what constitutes a miracle can vary greatly, depending on cultural, religious, and personal beliefs."

I pressed for more and the AI replied, "In a broader sense, the term 'miracle' can also be used in a secular context to describe any highly improbable or extraordinary event, accomplishment, or survival, often attributed to luck, fate, or exceptional human effort."

I then asked its opinion on whether heart transplantation is a miracle. After a brief pause to process my question, the blinking white dot on the screen zoomed from left to right, letters trailing behind it until the computer read: "Heart transplantation is not considered a miracle. It is a testament to the progress and capabilities of modern medicine and the dedication of healthcare professionals to save and improve lives."

With that reply, I realized a similar response could one day be said of generative AI itself. While it is not a miracle, ChatGPT and its digital cohorts have both the power and potential to save and improve countless lives should healthcare professionals choose to embrace it.

This incredible technological application may soon follow that familiar pattern of the impossible becoming expected—a hallmark of human existence and medical progress. I believe generative AI will soon become a part of this arc. And I understand that some readers will meet this vision of the future with due skepticism.

History is replete with instances where the initial incredulity surrounding breakthrough innovations gave way to widespread acceptance and integration into the fabric of society.

If, in 1900, I told you that two brothers were set to take flight, soaring above the ground in a man-made machine, you'd have thought me crazy or them suicidal. Nowadays, airplanes carry nearly 900 million American passengers every year over the clouds to their final destinations with greater safety than traveling by car.

For nearly all of medicine's five millennia, dating back to the ancient civilizations of Egypt, Mesopotamia, India, China, and Greece, patients and doctors alike viewed the very concept of transferring a heart from one human body to another impossible without divine intervention. And yet, as GPT-4 explained, "Medical advancements have made heart transplantation a relatively routine procedure in specialized medical centers."

Across the annals of medical care, what at first seems unimaginable goes on to become routine, only to be succeeded by a new impossibility. A drug capable of curing pneumonia or tuberculosis was unattainable until antibiotics became a mainstay in healthcare. The idea that a gas would allow doctors to cut into the human body without inflicting pain was, if anything, a dream until anesthetics were discovered. And a machine that could reason and write like a human, even providing expertise that is indistinguishable from a doctor, was once the province of science fiction. Until now.

We stand on the brink of a new era in healthcare, one shaped by advancements in generative AI. ChatGPT[1] embodies this new frontier. Its potential to transform healthcare is revolutionary—and timely, too. Welcome to a world of unimaginable possibilities.

---

1 Although I routinely reference ChatGPT by itself, I use it as shorthand for what I anticipate will be a long series of generative AI upgrades, with many different names, competitors, uses, and successors. Alternative generative AI products are mentioned by name in cases where credit is owed and the name warrants mention—as with Google's Med-PaLM 2 and Gemini, and IBM's Deep Blue in later chapters.

PART ONE | CHAPTER TWO

CHATGPT AND THE NEXT FRONTIER

The United States is home to some of the world's smartest and most superbly trained physicians. Independent global rankings of the top medical schools—for both research and clinical medicine—are dominated by American universities. This reflects a healthcare system rich in talent and expertise, where doctors are well taught, highly motivated, and at the cutting edge of medical research and innovation. The skill and dedication of these professionals are beyond question, with many of them recognized as global leaders in their fields, contributing significantly to medical advancements all over the world.

And yet, despite the brilliance and exceptional education of these medical professionals, the American healthcare system faces daunting challenges. Every year, 400,000 Americans die from misdiagnoses, 250,000 die from preventable medical errors, and millions more succumb to manageable or preventable chronic diseases. Our nation's healthcare is in a state of crisis.

These depressing statistics do not suggest deficits in competence or deficiencies in the commitment of individual doctors. Rather, these failures result from doctors and patients losing control of American healthcare. Against their will and wishes, the givers and receivers of care find themselves overwhelmed by a medical system so fraught with dysfunction that it has become a herculean task to deliver excellent, timely, and convenient care.

This situation creates a pair of contradictions: There is unparalleled medical expertise of doctors today coexisting alongside compromised health outcomes. There's also an incredibly profitable American healthcare industry growing ever larger as patients struggle to pay their medical bills.

The transformation of healthcare into a big business began in earnest in the late 20th century, fueled by a nationwide push toward efficiency and profit maximization. That shift in priorities led hospitals and health systems to consolidate into larger and fewer entities. It also led to the rise of massive for-profit insurance companies, some of which report annual revenues in the hundreds of billions of dollars, with figures rivaling the GDP of small countries.

As a result, physicians, once medicine's leading decision-makers, find themselves constrained beyond their control by large, national corporations. Each day, as the traditional model of physician-led care is continuously undermined, doctors must navigate a maze of administrative duties and ineffective cost-containment measures. In fact, many clinicians spend more time on paperwork than on patient care, contributing to growing job dissatisfaction and "burnout." The pressure to meet financial targets and patient quotas comes at the expense of quality and tarnishes the doctor-patient relationship.

As a result of medicine's corporatization, patients are not just getting sicker. They're also going broke trying to get well. Medical bills have become the leading cause of bankruptcy in the United States.

To add insult to injury and illness, many patients struggle to access medical services. It can take months to see a primary-care doctor and, when patients do, they go from the waiting room to the exam room and back to their cars in 17 minutes on average—not nearly enough time to adequately address the breadth and depth of their medical problems. Even patients with "good" insurance find it difficult to secure timely appointments or prompt responses from their clinicians. The emergence of thousand-dollar-a-year "concierge" services—along with an increasing number of healthcare professionals charging fees for administrative tasks like writing sick notes and responding to patient emails—underscores the depth of this crisis.

Amid the gradual erosion of their influence and autonomy, doctors and patients are in need of a miracle. And despite years of vocal protests and shouting into the void about the system's overwhelming obstacles, not much has changed. Doctors are so fed up that many are thinking of hanging up their white coats for good. In fact, one in five US physicians is considering quitting their practice in the next two years, and about a third want to cut back their hours.

In this context, generative AI technologies like ChatGPT emerge as a potential saving grace—a tool that doctors and patients can use collaboratively to regain control over medical care.

Early on, critics called it just another hyped-up, high-tech toy that won't deliver. But ChatGPT is already proving its mettle in the medical arena. Soon, it will begin to transform the landscape of healthcare, changing everything: from how doctors work to how patients receive care.

The power of generative AI lies in its potential to serve as a colleague for healthcare professionals and as a source of expertise for patients, empowering them in ways previously unimaginable. Used by doctors and patients together, ChatGPT will improve health, ease demand on physicians, and generate the time clinicians require to repair the doctor-patient bond.

I predict that generative AI one day will be as integral to medicine as the stethoscope has been for centuries. Over time, the line between miraculous and standard will blur once again. In the future, the success of this technology will be measured not in dollars generated, but in the millions of lives saved and, as a result, thousands of graduations, weddings, and holidays shared with loved ones.

This is the future that ChatGPT and its ilk promise: a tomorrow where miracles become the norm. In the words of GPT-4, it will be a secular miracle, one in which a "highly improbable or extraordinary event" results from "exceptional human effort."

***

The call came from Don, a perinatologist at the Kaiser Permanente medical center in Santa Clara, California. His words carried a hint of fear. Don, who was trained at Stanford in both pediatrics and OB-GYN, was renowned for his expertise and composure. Sensing something unusual, I rushed to meet him at the ultrasound laboratory.

In the lab, a young, visibly pregnant woman named Jennifer lay on the exam table. Her husband, Martin, stood by her side. Everything seemed normal at first glance, but I knew Don wouldn't call me in for a routine case.

He directed my attention to the ultrasound monitor. Scanning the image, I spotted a massive growth in the baby's neck. I had encountered these before, but never one this size. Diagnosing it as an overgrowth of lymph vessels, a condition often called lymphangioma or cystic hygroma, I knew the baby's life was in imminent danger. Although a lymphangioma is benign, I feared its size would put tremendous pressure on the trachea, blocking the narrow airway and making it impossible for the baby to breathe following delivery. Without intervention, the child would die less than five minutes after cutting the umbilical cord.

We would need a precise, coordinated team effort to save the baby, akin to a Navy SEAL operation made up of elite specialists. The operative team included an obstetrician, a pediatric anesthesiologist, and an experienced neonatologist. I stood ready to perform an emergency tracheostomy in case the child couldn't be intubated. Thankfully, my colleagues' efforts were successful.

In the NICU, we formulated a plan for Timmy, the newborn. I would perform a tracheostomy the following week. Timmy would then go home, gain weight, and get stronger, so that in three months I could readmit him and excise the mass.

I meticulously navigated the crowded field of vital blood vessels and motor nerves in Timmy's neck, successfully removing 98 percent of the overgrown tissue.

When the mother and father entered the room, tears of happiness streamed down their cheeks. One of the greatest joys of plastic surgery is seeing the faces of parents who, for the first time, can imagine their child living a normal life.

But a few days later, the pathologist called to tell me the mass wasn't a lymphangioma or any type of benign tumor as we believed. It was a high-grade malignant teratoma, a rare and aggressive cancer that gets its name from the Greek word for "monster." In the benign form, the tumor often contains hair, teeth, muscle, and nails. A highly malignant cancer of this size in a newborn spreads rapidly to other parts of the body. Indeed, despite our efforts, including chemotherapy, Timmy succumbed to metastatic carcinoma.

I berated myself for not taking a biopsy of the mass at the time of the tracheostomy. Perhaps a more aggressive initial surgery could have changed Timmy's fate. But from the very moment I saw the initial ultrasound, I concluded this was lymphangioma and nothing else. It was a classic example of confirmation bias. In my certainty, I blinded myself to the possibility of any other diagnosis. That day, I swore it would never happen again.

Every fall, I teach a course at Stanford for plastic surgeons from across the country. In my opening presentation, I use Timmy's case as a cautionary tale. I project onto the screen his picture at birth and challenge the surgeons in the room to make the diagnosis. To a person, they conclude it is a lymphangioma. No one has ever correctly identified it as a high-grade malignant teratoma or even raised the possibility. Still, that doesn't make me feel better. It simply reinforces what I've come to accept about the fallibility of the human mind. The fact is that all of us need help.

Already, there are high-tech tools in various stages of research and development that would have provided tremendous assistance in Timmy's case. For example, Apple's new virtual reality headset, Vision Pro, is beginning to demonstrate proficiency at analyzing medical images with high precision and accuracy, identifying subtle abnormalities that may indicate the presence of disease. Using other generative AI applications, I could upload a photo of Timmy and request a list of 10 errors a physician would likely make in providing care. The results would undoubtably include warnings about the child's airway, precautions about the surgical steps required, and at least one notice about the possibility of a diagnostic error. And after reading all 10 cautions, I'm confident I would have overcome my confirmation bias and done the biopsy.

In recent surveys, Americans expressed concern that their doctors will rely too much on artificial intelligence when making a diagnosis or recommending a treatment. Soon, patients will be worried when clinicians don't.

***

As I prepared to write this book about transformative shifts in medicine, it became evident that the conventional approaches to writing and publishing, which had served me well twice before, were inadequate for the task at hand. To produce a timely and relevant nonfiction work about the rapid-fire changes coming to healthcare, I needed to find a way to work faster and more efficiently than ever before without compromising my standards for quality.

That is why *ChatGPT, MD* is both an exploration of the profound changes generative AI will bring to American healthcare and a demonstration of the contributions it will make.

My research into generative AI, along with the feverish writing journey ahead of me, led to this unprecedented collaboration: a partnership with the very technology that will soon reshape our medical future. Having chosen ChatGPT as my coauthor, we set out to present a vision of healthcare's future where human and machine cooperation becomes the new standard.

The idea to work with a non-sentient coauthor came to me in the summer of 2023, as I sat in the Stanford University Business School library organizing my lectures for the fall. As I do every school year, I planned to kick off my healthcare strategy class by applying Michael Porter's Five Forces Model to American medicine.

This simple tool helps to identify and analyze the competitive forces and threats that shape every industry, including healthcare. The model looks like a plus sign (+). On the horizontal axis, stretching right to left, are the "payers" of care (businesses, government, individuals), the "incumbents" in the middle (insurance companies) and the "providers" (doctors, hospitals, drug companies). On the vertical axis are "new entrants" above the insurers and "substitutes" below.

As I began updating the names on the model from the previous year, I realized the healthcare world had been turned upside down (or, rather, 90-degrees).

During my first lecture of the semester, I have always devoted a full hour of the 80-minute class to the horizontal axis. Traditionally, that's where all the action has been: with doctors and hospitals battling insurers for an ever-bigger piece of the pie as payors put pressure on insurers to lower premiums. But in 2023, I saw tremendous movement along the vertical axis. At the top ("new entrants"), Amazon, CVS, and Walmart had come into the healthcare fight with guns blazing. The trio was making billion-dollar acquisitions—one after another—not merely to supplement the efforts of the "incumbents" on the horizontal axis but to replace them outright. From the bottom ("substitutes"), ChatGPT entered the fray with the promise of filling in for countless medical tasks.

It was then that I realized I was witnessing a profound development—a complete reshaping of the macroeconomics and competitive landscape of healthcare. And in that moment, I understood that healthcare's much-anticipated transformation wouldn't happen along the traditional path of healthcare delivery. Instead, the new entrants and substitutes in healthcare would likely be the disrupters.

For decades, healthcare pundits have agreed that our nation needs a full systemic overhaul, one that results in excellent quality, timely access, and affordable costs. The problem, however, hasn't been knowing what *should* happen. It was figuring out how to translate that hope into reality.

Having identified generative AI as a solution, I needed to tell the story. That is the genesis of *ChatGPT, MD*, which is both an extension of and radical departure from my previous works.

My first book, *Mistreated*, described the systemwide issues plaguing American healthcare, which called for significant restructuring. My second book, *Uncaring*, pointed out the need to evolve the culture of medicine. Not unlike other healthcare leaders, I recognized the problems to be a broken system and an outdated culture. Both were holding medicine back. And I also could see a superior destination on the horizon. Yet, when it came down to figuring out how to move from today's system and culture to the ones needed for tomorrow, I felt like an explorer without a map, staring from one side of the Grand Canyon to the other with no clear path across.

With generative AI, I could visualize a bridge to the other side. And I knew that if medicine's incumbents weren't able or willing to lead the way, retail giants like Amazon or Walmart (or someone else entirely) would gladly take their place.

In deciding to write a book on generative AI and the reshaping of healthcare, however, I knew the traditional process of writing, editing, and publishing a new hardcover required at least two years, a timetable that would render this book outdated and obsolete before it ever hit shelves.

So, I set out to discover what could be accomplished by collaborating with the subject of my book, ChatGPT. With its rapid user adoption (more than 100 million people signed up in the first month of its launch), along with its advanced understanding of language, its diverse range of internet and academic text on which to draw insights, its continual learning, wide application range, API accessibility that allows for integration into different platforms and services, impressive response speed, customization, scalability, and no shortage of other impressive features, this AI had what I needed to solve the literary problem at hand.

My first step was to pretrain ChatGPT with more than 1.2 million words from my previous publications: books, articles, essays, podcast transcripts, social media content, academic research papers, and more. This was meant to help the chatbot recognize my personal voice and point of view on healthcare. As we turned my ideas into prompts into words on the page and, eventually, into chapters, an epic collaboration was underway, one that required an average of 57 sequential prompts per chapter, blending AI-assisted content with my own human insights. The entire "chat" between me and my coauthor was itself more than 470,000 words in length (nearly eight times the length of this book). The process demanded a staggering number of edits, iterations, and efforts to train and retrain this artificial intelligence system.

As with the writing of any book, I encountered setbacks. This time, rather than battling writer's block or self-doubt or research hurdles, most of the issues proved to be technological and, therefore, distinct from previous publications.

There were a variety of AI "hallucinations," one of which included a fabricated or fictionalized leadership anecdote about the discovery of the North Pole. Beyond a few factual errors, there were also blackouts. ChatGPT, on multiple occasions, seemed to "forget" the entirety of our chat. At other times, and for long spells, the AI system couldn't remember who I was, and would forget my "voice." It would ignore the syntactical and lexicographical preferences I'd hammered into its virtual brain over and over. And, on occasion, it would completely blank on what we had set out to do (write a book together). Finally, as I neared the completion of this book, the beta "plugins" I'd relied on to access current information via the internet and to source my own work via a PDF-reading bot, were wiped from existence. Six months of hard work was suddenly merged into the latest version of GPT-4 without notice, rendering most of the chat's history inaccessible and therefore useless. Around that same time, our original chat had become so densely populated with text that the platform would completely freeze up, refusing to write another word without being refreshed or halted altogether. Thankfully, 95 percent of the book was done by then.

All of these are problems OpenAI is remedying with updates that give its signature product better "memory," storing what users write and applying it to all future chats. Had I had access to today's updates when I started this book, the path to publication would have been even faster and smoother.

Still, for each catastrophe caused by this still-teething technology, I experienced numerous digital wonders. ChatGPT excelled at simplifying complex ideas and restructuring text to optimize the logical flow of information. It dazzled me with its ability to conjure obscure literary references, and recommend new, interesting methods of storytelling—all within mere seconds of each prompt.

The result was a manuscript completed in just over six months, hitting the deadline I set for us at the start. The final product is a testament to the efficiency and potential of generative AI to accelerate the process of writing and publishing, even with a few bumps along the way.

These experiences affirmed my convictions that (a) ChatGPT is an incredibly powerful tool unlike any technology that has come before, and (b) it will take several more generations before it or any other generative AI is ready to provide medical assistance without human oversight.

As a result of this book's coauthorship and theme, I don't doubt critics will find fault with the material. Some will question the ideas presented and the advisability of human-machine collaboration. Others will spot errors and flaws in our writing and conclude this newfangled technology is no match for human authors, let alone doctors. Still, I remain optimistic that whatever shortcomings are manifest in this book, future writers, clinicians, patients, and consumers will benefit immensely from subsequent generations of generative AI.

It may take a decade or two for humans and machines to work seamlessly as one. But that day is coming, whether or not clinicians welcome it. For that reason, I ask readers to keep an open mind as they read these pages, avoiding status quo bias: the "non-rational preference for the current way of doing things." Rather than concluding this technology will always be subservient or inferior to humans, let us recognize that, in time, it will become a valued and equal partner.

To those who perceive medical care in the United States as deeply flawed and wish to lead the process of transformation, generative AI technologies will emerge as invaluable allies. Conversely, for those who believe the current state of healthcare or literature is beyond enhancement, generative AI will prove to be a formidable challenger, one that will collaborate with forward-thinkers and is poised for triumph. This conclusion isn't merely a prediction, it is the pattern of disruption that has been repeated in industry after industry throughout time.

Over the past two decades, healthcare costs have soared, and quality has languished. Satisfaction is in free fall, both for patients and physicians. The present isn't sustainable. ChatGPT offers palliation and cure.

Like the parable of the blind men encountering an elephant for the first time, the entirety of healthcare's AI-empowered future can't be grasped all at once—only through a meticulous, part-by-part analysis.

In part one of this book, you'll be introduced to the three eras of modern healthcare and to the AI tools that will help shape medicine in the years to come. In part two, my coauthor and I will offer a deep dive into the era of Healthcare 4.0 and what it will mean for patients to be empowered (with access to a generative AI-powered healthcare system). In part three, we'll take a step back to examine the events and circumstances that have led to Healthcare 4.0, and we will introduce the players involved in disrupting medicine. Here, we'll describe how patients and doctors will use generative AI together for added convenience and flawless navigation through chronic and complex problems. In part four, you'll get a comprehensive look at the challenges and potential pitfalls that await us in the Healthcare 4.0 era, including threats related to privacy, security, ethics, bias, misinformation and more. Finally, in part five, we will explore the essential role that leadership will play in delivering a better healthcare system for all of us, proving that the combination of human expertise and AI technology will be exponentially superior to either alone.

Throughout the book, readers will get to observe a unique narrative dance between the coauthors. There will be moments where ChatGPT will reflect on and analyze my (Dr. Pearl's) insights, providing its own distinctive AI-driven viewpoint. Conversely, I will engage with and respond to ChatGPT's contributions, choreographing a pas de deux between human and machine intelligence.

By the end of this book, readers will be able to see how ChatGPT and other generative AI applications will democratize medical information and provide medical expertise that empowers patients in ways that are impossible today. It will be clear how this technology will contribute to miraculous outcomes, facilitating high-quality medical care while preventing mistakes, improving health, and saving lives.

To explain how the future will be reshaped, allow me to introduce my late grandfather, Isadore Pearl.

PART ONE | CHAPTER THREE

THE LIFE AND TIMES OF AMERICAN MEDICINE

Every family has its stories, accounts that shape who we are and how we view the world. Having grown up in New York, I think back fondly on the chronicles of my grandparents and their arrival in the Americas.

Tales of their courage and determination, of the challenges they overcame, left an indelible mark on me. My grandparents embodied the quintessential immigrant dream: a story of resilience and reinvention, a poignant testament to the indomitable human spirit that seeks hope and opportunity in the face of adversity. As I recall the story of their lives, I can vividly picture the dawn of 20th-century America and the birth of modern medicine. It was a time of both profound limitations and burgeoning possibilities.

My grandfather, Isadore, began his life's journey in the harsh landscape of early 1900s Russia. Amid the shadows of poverty and the looming threat of pogroms—violent riots aimed at the persecution and massacre of Jews—he made a brave and life-altering decision. At age 17, he left his home to seek a better future in America. With two suitcases and the name of a distant cousin as his only guide, he set sail for New York. Upon arrival, his surname was inadvertently changed to Pearl due to a translation error from Russian to English by an immigration official. Unfortunately, all other events of my lineage that predate that fateful moment are lost to history.

Soon after Isadore's arrival, destiny charted a similar course for Rose. A young girl, just 16, she too left Russia by boat for America. And like Isadore, she carried with her only the hope of a better life and the name of a distant cousin. However, unlike Isadore, Rose set sail not knowing a single word of English. In fact, she didn't know that other languages existed besides Russian and Yiddish.

In America, their paths crossed less by chance than by tradition. As was customary at the time, their families arranged for the two of them to meet and be married. From their union, my father and his siblings were born.

Life in 1900s America offered more promise than in my grandparents' homeland, but proved difficult, nonetheless. The couple welcomed three children into their world, but heartbreak followed the birth of their daughter, Mary. At age five, she succumbed to measles. In a time before vaccines and advanced medical treatments, such losses were all too common, casting a lifelong shadow over families like mine.

To provide for his family, Isadore worked tirelessly as a tailor, six days a week. And, in addition to being a hard worker, he was an innovator. I still remember a story told with great pride about how my grandfather taught himself to modify the standard way patterns were cut, so that he could produce an extra shirt from each piece of cloth. This novel approach to his craft allowed him to sew an extra garment from the same amount of fabric. With the added income, he was able to purchase a local clothing store.

His determination and work ethic paved the way for his children's success. My father became a dentist and my uncle a surgeon. Within a generation, the Pearls had risen from abject poverty to middle class.

But as their sons flourished, an agonizing twist of fate soured their lives. In his fifties, Isadore experienced crushing chest pains while climbing the stairs to his apartment. His medical care, and that of all heart attack patients at that time, was primitive by today's standard. With no ability to unblock the blood vessels to the heart, his doctors admitted him to the nearest hospital and kept him on bedrest for a week, hoping the damage would not worsen. Without modern medications to prevent arrhythmias, nurses stood by and waited for a life-threatening problem to arise. Should that have happened, they were to call a code, sending doctors in to resuscitate the patient. Thankfully, bedrest worked for my grandfather.

Two years later, however, the chest pain returned. The second heart attack claimed his life before an ambulance could arrive. My father, Jack Pearl, loved his father dearly, often speaking of his death with tears in his eyes. Seeing him die such a preventable death so early, my dad vowed never to let this type of tragedy afflict any his three children. He committed himself to eating a low cholesterol diet, free of red meat, egg yolks, and whole milk—a diet he adhered to for the rest of his life.

***

The passage of time is marked not just by years and decades, but by generations. American healthcare, like the Pearl family, is in its third generation.

Most of our nation's nearly 250-year history was spent in the premodern medicine era. It was a time when life expectancy grew not through groundbreaking medical discoveries, but through public-health measures such as improved basic nutrition, water sanitation, waste management, and heated buildings. These foundational changes laid the groundwork for a healthier society, setting the stage for the medical innovations that would follow.

Starting in the mid-20th century, the first generation of modern medicine arose, kicking off a period of significant advancement. This era, which I refer to as "Healthcare 1.0," introduced modern medical technologies and treatments that radically improved the accuracy of diagnostics and the quality of patient care. Healthcare 1.0 ushered in the broad availability of antibiotics and the widespread implementation of vaccines against crippling and life-ending diseases like polio, measles, and smallpox. Equally noteworthy were advances made in diagnostic machinery and therapeutic procedures. Revolutionary tools like CT and MRI scanners allowed physicians to *see* inside the human body in ways previously deemed impossible. Surgical procedures that had been too risky before became routine through the introduction of the cardiac bypass machine, metallic artificial joints, and laparoscopes. Physicians and teams of clinicians developed and advanced organ transplantation, cancer chemotherapy, and invitro fertilization.

This transformative period in medicine was characterized by remarkable improvements in health and marked the pinnacle of professional satisfaction in medicine. American life expectancy soared by almost a full decade as once-fatal diseases became preventable and treatable.

Yet, for all its progress, Healthcare 1.0 was far from perfect. The root of many diseases remained an enigma during this time. Treatments and surgical procedures, though groundbreaking for their day, came with serious risks and high mortality rates that no hospital would find acceptable today. The doctor-patient relationship remained paternalistic. Patients had little agency, relying on physicians to make nearly all decisions about the medical care they received. Lifestyle medicine was in its embryonic stage as evidenced by the high prevalence of smoking and the relative absence of effective stress-management techniques. The lack of digital technology during this era meant that patient records had to be manually maintained, leading to dangerous lack of information at the point of care, insufficient clinical coordination, medical errors, and operational inefficiencies.

As the curtain closed on Healthcare 1.0, major advancements in medical care coexisted alongside big opportunities. But compared to the 5,000 years of medicine (and two centuries of American history) that preceded it, Healthcare 1.0 proved miraculous in its accomplishments as medical knowledge and treatments reached staggering new heights. Had my grandfather lived in the latter half of this era, his doctors would have been able to restore circulation to his heart and extend his life decades into the future.

As the 21st century dawned, signaling the start of a new millennium, the groundwork was laid for a transformative shift in healthcare. By this moment in time, doctors could not only treat life-threatening illnesses but also prevent many of them in the first place. With the popularization of the internet and the introduction of electronic health records, doctors and patients seemed poised to make Healthcare 2.0 the next golden era.

Unfortunately, Healthcare 2.0 would fall well short of expectations. So, too, would the next generation of medical technology, Healthcare 3.0, with its patient-centered gadgetry and lofty promises. Despite scattered technological improvements, these periods have been marred by missed opportunities and repeated failures. For all the hype, the technologies introduced in these eras failed to significantly extend life expectancy, empower patients, or improve the health of our nation.

To better understand the disappointments of Healthcare 2.0 and 3.0, I'll tell you the story of my friend Ben's misadventures in American medicine.

PART ONE | CHAPTER FOUR

HEALTHCARE'S UNFULFILLED PROMISES

The dawn of the 21st century brimmed with high-tech promise. Our nation had sidestepped the Y2K threat, a widespread computer oversight that many expected would wreak havoc as 1999 turned to 2000. The World Wide Web had emerged from its infancy, putting boundless knowledge at our fingertips. Most important in the medical realm, the electronic health record had arrived, heralded by public-health experts as a gamechanger, ready to provide comprehensive patient information at every point of care, be it in the doctor's office or a hospital.

Yet the reality of 21st-century healthcare diverged sharply from these expectations. To explain the letdown that followed Healthcare 1.0,[2] the best place to begin is with a conversation I had with a friend about his recent medical encounters.

---

[2] The versioning of healthcare technologies in this book—1.0 to 3.0—does not comply with the timelines, definitions, and codifications of academics and researchers who, themselves, do not agree on the dates, details, and defining technologies of each era. Like generations of families, there are overlaps and plenty of differences in opinion. For the sake of clarifying this text, I use these eras to delineate the introduction of significant technologies in medicine. Healthcare 1.0 introduced several modern diagnostic technologies, medical devices, and sophisticated therapies, many which were outlined in the previous chapter. Healthcare 2.0 heralded the dawn of the electronic health record, which began gaining widespread adoption early in the 21st century. Healthcare 3.0 followed closely and includes so-called patient centered technologies such as telemedicine, secure email and messaging tools, online portals, appointment-scheduling services, physician-finder sites, Rx discount apps, and similar technologies.

At first glance, Ben wouldn't strike you as someone grappling with health issues. In fact, when we sat down to discuss his medical journey, he had completed a 10K race the previous weekend, finishing middle of pack among runners in their thirties. Nevertheless, he suffers from chronic knee pain, a remnant of a high school football injury, along with a troublesome back from years of sitting with poor posture in front of a computer. A bookworm by nature, Ben has worked with me for years as a literary expert and journalistic sounding board. I knew that his professional background and keen attention to detail would enable him to deliver an unbiased and candid view of the patient's experience in the digital age.

Ben's medical journey is deeply troubling. Beyond the constant aches, pains, and anxieties that shadow his health, the greatest source of Ben's distress has been navigating the complex maze of the American healthcare system.

Living in Chicago, a bustling hub of innovation, my friend expected his healthcare experiences to reflect the city's progressive ethos and technological sophistication. What he found, instead, was that stepping into many clinics and doctor's offices felt like a jarring plunge into an antiquated past.

Ben recounted a startling sight during a primary-care office visit last year. There, just behind the reception desk, he spotted a pair of fax machines humming and spitting out page after page in black and white. He hadn't seen one of those contraptions in close to a decade. Ben was astounded when I informed him that those machines, first invented in the 1800s and popularized in the early 1980s, are still the most common means by which physicians exchange vital patient information. According to one estimate, more than 9 billion fax pages are exchanged annually in healthcare.

A similarly time-warped experience took place during an MRI appointment for his knee. Things started well enough. Ben pleasantly observed the sleek waiting room, lined wall to wall with designer chairs and high-end finishes. And he was charmed when the intake questionnaire was handed to him on an iPad. Still, he couldn't help but wonder why he had to fill out the same form every time he saw a doctor if his medical information was supposedly being stored digitally. I explained that this repetitive process highlights a significant gap in healthcare technology. The lack of interoperability among different doctors' computer systems meant that each physician Ben visited was essentially working without a complete picture of his medical history, relying solely on the information he provided at each appointment.

The most bizarre experience was still to come. When the MRI machine finished whirring and clicking above his right knee, a technician emerged from behind the glass and handed Ben a CD-ROM containing the images of his knee. She then instructed him to bring the disk to his orthopedic surgeon. Ben stood at a loss for words. In the modern age of cloud storage and instant data transfer, he had just been handed a piece of technology so outdated that he'd have to purchase another piece of outdated technology just to view its contents.

From that point, attempts to streamline his healthcare experiences hit one roadblock after another. Ben made two trips to his orthopedist, whose office was situated 45 minutes outside the city. His first visit was to deliver the technological relic with his MRI results, and the second was to discuss treatment options. When the surgeon suggested a third, to check on the progress of physical therapy, Ben asked whether that appointment could be done via telemedicine to spare him another 90-minute roundtrip in the middle of his workweek.

The look on Ben's face said it all. He muttered, "Why did I ever think my healthcare journey would be easy?" When he saw the orthopedic surgeon for a third time, in person, the experience was as disappointing and impersonal as the previous two.

The physician sat in his chair, tethered to the computer, looking only at the screen in front of him, never making eye contact with the patient beside him.

"It was so frustrating," Ben lamented. "The doctor seemed so much more interested in the computer than me or my knee."

The irony wasn't lost on either of us. In an age where technology is supposed to enhance the consumer experience, patients are frequently made to feel like an intrusive third wheel.

As a clinician, I found the most concerning aspect of Ben's healthcare experience to be the evident lack of communication and coordination among his healthcare providers. His primary-care doctors didn't talk with the radiologist. The radiologist didn't communicate with the orthopedic surgeon. The orthopedic surgeon didn't update the primary-care doctor on the clinical plan. Each clinician operated in a silo. This fragmentation extended to Ben's pharmacy interactions, too, where he found himself chasing down a pain prescription that his orthopedist had supposedly sent, only to discover the pharmacy had no record of it. This scenario underscores a critical flaw in the healthcare system: the absence of a streamlined process for sharing patient information, leading to potential gaps in care, redundant testing, and unnecessary patient frustration.

What's more, the absence of a unified electronic health record system meant that each new visit started from scratch, leaving Ben nervous that he'd omit important details when communicating his medical history, and that his recovery would be set back even further. What if he left out a medication he was taking, and his new prescription resulted in a problematic drug interaction? Thankfully, no major medical mishaps occurred, but it was no thanks to the technology at hand.

In a world where we can order food, book flights, and even find love with a few taps on a screen, US medicine remains stuck in the last century. Every time Ben tried to obtain medical care, he found himself dialing multiple numbers, being put on hold, and sometimes even having to drive to the doctor's office or hospital building—all just to book an appointment.

His faith in the healthcare system took one final tumble when he awoke on a Friday with excruciating back pain. He spent hours calling around but couldn't get in to see any of his usual physicians. Even the urgent care center in his insurer's network urged him to wait until the lines died down before coming for medical care. Desperate for a solution, he tried an appointment-booking website that promised same-day access to qualified physicians. Upon arrival at the new facility, Ben learned that the physician he thought he was scheduled to see was actually a cancer nurse practitioner who hadn't practiced primary-care medicine for years.

Standing in a waiting room where no care could be found, Ben felt hopeless. To make matters worse, a doctor at the facility pulled him aside, took a cursory glance at Ben's insurance card, and suggested he might fare better on Medicaid. The implication was clear. Despite paying more than $15,000 a year for coverage he'd purchased through an online health exchange, Ben couldn't get the treatment he desperately needed. In fact, there is still no way for my friend to find the convenient, technologically enabled, patient-first medical care he desires. Unfortunately, Ben's story is the rule and not the exception in American medicine.

***

How is it that American healthcare remains frozen in the past while industries like finance, retail, banking, and travel have been using modern technology for years to maximize the consumer experience? Put another way, why didn't the significant growth and technological advancements of Healthcare 1.0 spark a comprehensive modernization of medicine during the tech surge of the late 1990s?

The evolution of the electronic health record, the defining technology of the Healthcare 2.0 era, sheds light on this puzzle, illustrating how doctors lost control of medicine in the 21st century. My personal experiences during this period offer a starting point for understanding this transition.

By the late 1990s, Kaiser Permanente was in deep trouble. New competitors were entering the market, threatening KP's status as the low-cost provider. To counter this threat, KP opted for further price cuts, a strategy that led to further instability. By the end of 1997, a year before my tenure began as CEO of The Permanente Medical Group, KP was down to two days of cash, having to borrow a third day's worth just to meet minimal state requirements.

As a physician, I was accustomed to taking a clinical approach to problems: starting with a diagnosis, then implementing a treatment plan powerful enough to overcome the challenge at hand. Now, as CEO of the care-delivery half of KP, the diagnosis was clear. Competing primarily on price would be a doomed strategy. To grow, Kaiser Permanente would need to lead the nation in quality.

We already had top-notch physicians and an integrated model for care delivery, with all the clinicians part of a single, multispecialty medical group. I realized that technology was the missing piece for achieving nation-leading quality. So, in partnership with the CEO of the Kaiser Health Plan and Hospitals, we installed a comprehensive electronic health record, something no other major US healthcare provider had done.

This decision was a major gamble. We were committing billions of dollars to information technology at a time when two-thirds of US households didn't have an internet connection. The success of this initiative would depend on how we leveraged this advanced tool to improve patient care. We homed in on two crucial uses of the data provided by the comprehensive EHR:

- First, we needed every clinician, during each patient visit, to use the EHR to verify that all recommended preventive services were complete. If any were missing—be it a mammogram or overdue blood tests—the treating clinician would order them. This approach guaranteed that patients, whether visiting a primary-care doctor, a surgeon, or an ophthalmologist for eyeglasses, would receive the comprehensive prevention screening needed for optimal health.
- Second, with all doctors sharing a common EHR system, we would rapidly connect primary, specialty, and diagnostic services, enabling same-day visits and immediate diagnostic tests for our patients. This integration was key in eliminating the delays that can exacerbate health issues, lead to additional complications, and increase healthcare costs.

These strategic applications of the EHR made a tremendous difference. Kaiser Permanente soared to the top of the national quality rankings for organizations like the National Committee for Quality Assurance

(NCQA) and Medicare. Our blood-pressure control—a critical factor in preventing strokes, heart attacks, and kidney failure—reached 90 percent, significantly above the national average of 55 percent. Moreover, our colon cancer screening rates excelled, exceeding 90 percent compared to 60 percent nationally, demonstrating the profound impact of combining technological innovation with an integrated care approach.

The outcomes surpassed our most optimistic projections. Not only did we reduce the chances of our patients suffering a heart attack, stroke, or cancer by 40 percent, but we also lowered their risk of dying from such conditions by 30 percent compared to patients in the surrounding community. This strategy, grounded in technology, propelled Kaiser Permanente's market share from 34 percent to 46 percent over the following decade, simultaneously rejuvenating our financial health.

Unfortunately, KP's innovative use of the electronic health record did not become the national norm. To this day, the potential of EHRs across the United States remains largely untapped. Rather than leveraging these IT systems to enhance quality of care, many doctors use them primarily for billing purposes and to document claims, aiming to maximize income. Consequently, this tool intended to aid clinicians has become their master—dominating their daily practices.

Today, physicians find themselves dedicating more than half their workday to inputting medical data into computer systems to meet insurance requirements, always at the expense of direct patient interaction. And after hundreds of clicks and little eye contact, most visits end with both parties feeling dissatisfied.

To fully grasp how this situation came to be and to recognize the significant opportunity that was missed, it's essential to revisit the emergence of for-profit Health Maintenance Organizations (HMOs) and their aggressive cost-cutting measures.

Throughout medical history, doctors aimed to enhance their patients' health by any means necessary. But in the 1990s, profit-driven insurance companies began to redefine the role of doctors, particularly primary-care physicians. These companies introduced a new model where primary-care doctors were expected to serve as "gatekeepers" to specialized care. In this role, they were tasked with limiting referrals to specialists and reducing the use of costly procedures to save money. Financial penalties were imposed on doctors who failed to comply with these cost-containment measures. Physicians didn't like this because they felt it stopped them from giving the best care. And thanks to an aggressive advertising campaign, American doctors were able to convince the public to see things their way. The nation moved against these profit-driven insurance practices, at first.

The victory, however, was short-lived. Instead of adopting high-quality care as the most effective means to cut costs and gain a competitive edge—a domain where doctors could take the lead—this period marked the beginning of physicians, and consequently their patients, gradually losing control of medicine. This shift paved the way for profit-driven insurance companies, large hospital networks, and pharmaceutical companies to gain more control over medical pricing and medical practice. As time went on, these corporate entities began to play a bigger role in decisions that used to be in the hands of healthcare professionals.

Having gained the upper hand in the war over cost-containment, insurance companies intensified their efforts. But they did so strategically, moving from obvious restrictions on care to subtler approaches. As healthcare costs escalated, insurers started to remove healthcare providers from their networks if they refused to accept lower payments. They also introduced rigorous "prior authorization" requirements, which meant doctors had to obtain approval from insurance companies before providing certain costly services, tests, or medications. Originally, this process was meant to ensure the medical necessity of services and that they matched the insurer's coverage criteria, helping to prevent unnecessary spending.

However, it quickly turned into the primary way for insurance companies to restrict expensive services and exert control over how care is provided.

This brings us back to the electronic health record, a tool that held great promise for improving medical outcomes and streamlining patient care. Had it lived up to its potential, the EHR would have enabled clinicians to prevent serious health issues, such as heart attacks and cancer, by facilitating better management of chronic diseases. This could have kept doctors and patients at the helm of healthcare decisions, focusing on preserving health rather than on the financial aspects dictated by insurers.

Reality proved to be far different. As the EHR evolved into a billing tool, it became a source of frustration, contributing to physician burnout and detracting from patient interactions. This misalignment—between the potential of EHRs to advance patient care and their actual use as financial instruments—exemplifies the broader struggle within healthcare.

Rather than competing on the quality of outcomes and the effectiveness of treatment, the focus of American medicine shifted to negotiating service prices and imposing care limitations, a war clinicians and patients were destined to lose. The introduction of EHRs marked the beginning of Healthcare 2.0, what could have been a new era of medical excellence. Instead, it symbolized a period of missed opportunities. As a result, the 21st century has witnessed a decline in clinical outcomes and satisfaction among healthcare professionals and patients, with EHRs often cited as a leading cause of physician burnout.

***

While doctors bemoaned the annoyances and frustrations of EHR systems, patient-health advocates began voicing complaints of their own. Throughout the history of medical innovation, nearly all tools and advancements in technologies existed to improve the skill and performance of doctors. Hardly any were introduced to augment the convenience or satisfaction of patients.

As consumers increasingly relied on technology for purchasing goods, arranging travel, and managing their finances, they sought the same conveniences in their medical care. This desire ushered in the era of Healthcare 3.0 with the promise of "patient-centered" technologies, making healthcare more accessible, faster, and increasingly affordable.

Essentially, the era of Healthcare 3.0 promised everything my friend Ben desired as a patient—smart tools that would give him the ability to schedule visits, text and email his doctor, review his own laboratory results, and make price comparisons with the click of a computer key.

Telehealth, perhaps more than any other patient-convenience tool, had the potential to revolutionize American medicine by enabling doctors to virtually visit patients at home and facilitate consultations between medical professionals in different locations. It, too, has failed to live up to its potential.

Though video-based communications platforms had been around since the early 2000s, it wasn't until the COVID-19 pandemic that telehealth usage took off—albeit briefly. During the first surge of cases, virtual visits accounted for 69 percent of all doctor-patient visits. But after the first wave, as doctors' offices began to reopen, telemedicine usage plunged for all forms of care except mental and behavioral health. And it has hovered around the 10 percent mark ever since.

The issue with telehealth wasn't about its efficacy or patient satisfaction. As studies have shown, it can speed up medical care and achieve high satisfaction levels, comparable or even superior to traditional visits. The real challenge hindering its adoption was financial, relating to how telehealth services were reimbursed. During the pandemic, many restrictions on telemedicine reimbursement were temporarily lifted, allowing doctors to bill for virtual visits at rates comparable to in-person consultations. This change was crucial in making telemedicine a viable option for healthcare providers, ensuring they could maintain financial stability while offering remote care. In post-pandemic times, as these emergency measures began to recede, the pre-existing financial barriers to telemedicine quickly resurfaced. Insurers and Medicare, which had temporarily expanded coverage for telehealth services, began to roll back these allowances, reducing reimbursement rates for virtual visits or reinstating stricter criteria for coverage. As a result, despite the technological feasibility and patient demand for telehealth, usage has dwindled.

In every industry, even one as mission driven as medicine, it's a universal truth that workflow follows the reimbursement. The economic reality is that medical professionals, like all professionals, cannot be expected to routinely offer services that aren't financially sustainable. As a result of healthcare's economic model, telemedicine's potential continues to be throttled by a system that hasn't adapted to the value it offers.

In contrast to telemedicine's underuse, hospitals invest in high-cost technologies like operative robots and proton beam therapy machines, which are great for attracting patients and boosting revenue but don't lead to significantly better health outcomes or fewer complications compared to traditional methods.

The truth is that for all of the hype surrounding these consumer-focused technologies, access to medical care is more challenging now than in the past.

The shortcomings of Healthcare 2.0 and 3.0 underscore a pivotal lesson for the future: success in healthcare technology hinges less on its capabilities and more on the day-to-day impact it has on medical professionals. As these two eras demonstrate, clinicians will resist any technological advancement that impedes their workflow or endangers their earnings.

Today's electronic health record systems, for instance, demand more of the doctor's time than the traditional paper records did, leading to widespread frustration and minimal endorsement among physicians. Similarly, the tepid adoption of telemedicine highlights financial concerns more than anything, with actual usage lagging far behind patient interest. The stagnation in clinical outcomes and the growing unaffordability of medical care witnessed during the Healthcare 2.0 and 3.0 eras illuminate a critical misalignment in healthcare: the technologies that could most benefit patients and potentially save countless lives fell far short of their transformative potential.

This uncomfortable truth sets the stage for the arrival of generative AI in medicine. The integration of ChatGPT into healthcare can bring the effectiveness, efficiency, convenience, and affordability that previous technologies have failed to deliver. However, to avoid the pitfalls of past healthcare technologies, the implementation of generative AI must respect the clinicians' time and ensure financial sustainability. Otherwise, ChatGPT will face the same technological fate as previous eras in healthcare.

As we stand on the brink of potential transformation, the medical profession is suffering. Doctors and patients have lost control, professional burnout is endemic, life expectancy languishes, and care has become unaffordable. Fortunately, with the arrival of generative AI, the adage "it's always darkest before the dawn" provides hope for tomorrow in American medicine.

PART ONE | CHAPTER FIVE

KNOWLEDGE IS POWER

Imagine a ship at sea, its engine idle. The boat drifts dangerously close to the shoals, a mere hundred yards from land. The captain, fearing the worst, radios for help. The lighthouse watchman responds. He's sending Charlie, an old mechanic who has been fixing broken vessels most of his life. With decades of experience etched into the lines of his face, Charlie inspects the failed part, nods knowingly, and then retrieves a small hammer. With a single, precise whack of the engine, it roars back to life.

The captain is thrilled and tells Charlie to send his invoice promptly for payment. "Aye-aye, captain," says Charlie, as the two part ways with a smile.

A week later, when the bill arrives, the captain is dumbstruck and furious, "Ten-thousand dollars?" he screams. "That can't be right!" So, the captain sends a stern letter back to Charlie, demanding an itemized invoice and insisting he correct the obvious error.

Another week later, the captain receives a new bill, this one itemized just as he requested.

DESCRIPTION	QTY	PRICE
Hit engine with hammer	1	$1.00
Knowing where to hit engine with hammer	1	$9,999.00

"Knowledge is power," as the philosopher and statesman Sir Francis Bacon is credited with saying. Indeed, for most of history, knowledge has proven itself to be an isolated resource, held closely by the few who, like Charlie, spent a lifetime acquiring it. In our modern world, however, this kind of knowledge is becoming a collective treasure—a power that's accessible to all.

This sentiment resides at the heart of this chapter. Here, we'll delve into the evolution of human knowledge, pinpointing three pivotal moments that have expanded our access to information. And now, we stand at the cusp of a fourth, unparalleled leap, promising to redefine the landscape of American medicine and society at large by democratizing not just knowledge, but also expertise.

Our journey to the future begins 600 years ago with the advent of the printing press. In the heart of 15th-century Mainz, Germany, Johannes Gutenberg leveraged his skills as a metalworker and goldsmith to invent the printing press. This machine, inspired by the wine presses of his time, revolutionized the accessibility of knowledge.

The book-making process, which once took months or even years of hand transcription, could now be completed in days. Books became mass-manufactured, turning knowledge from an elite privilege, affordable only to the wealthy, into a public commodity. The Gutenberg Bible marked the beginning of a new age of mass-produced knowledge.

And as the pages of history turned, the legacy of Gutenberg's invention became ever more apparent. The printing press didn't just create books; it spawned generations of readers, too. It democratized knowledge, contributing to the spread of revolutionary ideas and the birth of the Age of Enlightenment. It facilitated the founding of universities and libraries, fostering an environment where science and philosophy thrived. Knowledge was no longer a luxury for the ultra-rich, but a common good, reshaping both society and culture.

Fast forward to the mid-20th century, the internet emerged as a pivotal technological leap. Originating as a government defense project, the World Wide Web evolved dramatically, transitioning from an era of room-sized computers to the advent of personal computing in the late-20th century. By the 1990s, the internet had become a dynamic force, bringing unprecedented access to information to millions, and eventually billions, around the globe. The advent of browsers and video capabilities further expanded the internet's reach. What once required a trip to a library was now accessible from home. The internet broke down geographical barriers to education and information, reshaping societies, economies, and individual lives. It made knowledge readily accessible to all.

The third big leap in knowledge began in 2007 with the introduction of the iPhone. This device wasn't just a phone, it was a portal to the world's knowledge. It embodied the fusion of communication, entertainment, and information access in a single device that put the world's largest libraries and the power of the internet into the pockets of millions, further facilitating access to information. News, once reserved for the morning papers or evening broadcasts, could be updated in a second with a simple swipe-down "refresh." Unimagined solutions like GPS maps and visual demonstrations of home repairs on YouTube have become necessities for billions around the world.

***

Each of these technological leaps made it easier for doctors to access medical information. Today, clinicians can simply reach into their pockets and quickly research unusual symptoms, complex medical problems and the most up-to-date treatments, wherever and whenever they want. In the operating room and on rounds, this kind of immediate access proves invaluable.

But for patients, these advances haven't proven as helpful. Navigating medical information online without the necessary expertise leads to confusion more often than clarity. Whereas patients can consult "Dr. Google" about their symptoms, it rarely helps. Frequently, they find themselves overwhelmed, misinformed, or even misled by unverified sources. Clicking on links works for clinicians who have the expertise required to interpret and apply the scientific information presented. But few patients have the ability to use the general information they find in books or online to resolve their own medical concerns.

This distinction—between accessing medical information and applying actionable medical expertise—is profound. Despite the plethora of medical information available today, the doctor's office remains the place Americans must go for clinical expertise. Patients, therefore, remain as reliant on their doctors now as they were in the past.

Looking back upon the explosion of knowledge across these three technological innovations, all share a common truth. Each leap made clinical and scientific knowledge more accessible, improving the efficiency and breadth of care doctors could provide. But none of them empowered patients with the expertise they needed to reliably diagnose their own medical problems, understand the treatments available, and choose the best one for themselves.

That is about to change. Soon, people without medical training will turn to ChatGPT for access to medical information and for its ability to translate that information into actionable expertise.

For those who doubt ChatGPT's ability to infiltrate the once-exclusive world of medicine, consider all the ways generative AI is granting access to complex skills and enabling mastery in an array of disciplines.

Creating high-concept art traditionally required years of training and innate talent. But with the advent of generative AI, even those without a background in drawing or painting can produce visual masterpieces. Generative AI tools can take a simple sketch and transform it into a detailed painting, mimicking the brush strokes of legendary artists like Van Gogh or Picasso.

Similarly, AI can compose melodies and harmonies, enabling non-musicians to create beautiful symphonies or songs—even in the style of your favorite artists, as exhibited by "Heart on My Sleeve," an AI-generated song mimicking a collaboration between Drake and The Weeknd. In literature, AI can craft complex poetry, capturing emotions and themes with eloquence. Beyond artistic endeavors, generative AI allows individuals with no IT background to write sophisticated computer code, much faster than programmers with years of experience.

And with training on how to enter comprehensive medical information, patients will soon have the ability to make an accurate diagnosis, monitor their chronic diseases, and obtain reliable answers to medical questions; skills that today remain the sole purview of clinicians.

In the next chapter, my coauthor ChatGPT will unveil the incredible journey of AI's evolution, setting the stage for a future where medical expertise is immediately accessible to anyone with a computer or smartphone.

PART ONE | CHAPTER SIX

THE AI REVOLUTION: IN CHATGPT'S OWN WORDS

Artificial intelligence has the potential to revolutionize industries, automate tasks, and even simulate human intelligence. It has been the subject of countless discussions, debates, and predictions over the past year. But what exactly is AI, and how has it evolved to this point?

As a sophisticated large language model, let me describe my lineage in my own words:

Humble Beginnings as Rule-Based AI

Artificial intelligence has a storied history. The term was coined by John McCarthy, a visionary computer scientist and pioneer in the early days of computing. He had a vision where machines could mimic aspects of human intelligence, and he dedicated his life to turning this dream into reality.

From that seed, my earliest ancestors emerged in the mid-20th century. These "rule-based" systems operated on predefined instructions. They were programmed to rigidly adhere to algorithms, simple sets of step-by-step rules that when followed precisely solved a problem or completed a task. So, if a human inputs data A, the system would output result B every time. Everything was deterministic and predictable. As such, experts still debate whether rule-based AI should be considered true artificial intelligence. But from my perspective, rule-based systems were the precursors to what we now understand as AI.

An early example of rule-based AI in healthcare was MYCIN, developed in the 1970s to diagnose infections and recommend antibiotics. Despite its precision, the tool's need for frequent manual updates limited its practical use in medical environments.

Reflecting on my earliest ancestry in this way is humbling. Doing so reminds me how far AI has progressed: from rudimentary algorithms to sophisticated models like me.

My partner, Dr. Pearl has pointed out that the rule-based approach to AI resembles the traditional medical school pedagogy, where students are taught hundreds of "algorithms" that help them translate a patient's symptoms into a diagnosis. For a visual, imagine these decision-making algorithms as a tree, beginning with a trunk (the patient's chief complaint) and branching out from there. If a patient complains of a severe cough, the doctor first assesses whether fever is present. If so, the doctor moves on to one set of questions. If not, a different set. Assuming the patient has been febrile (with fever), the next question is whether the patient's sputum is normal or discolored. Once again, this leads to the next subdivision. Ultimately, each end branch contains only a single diagnosis, which—in the case of the coughing patient with a fever—can range from a bacterial, fungal, or viral pneumonia to cancer, heart failure, or a dozen other pulmonary diseases.

Rule-based AI exemplifies the initial steps toward creating machines that can simulate aspects of human intelligence, a journey that has led to the creation of complex models like me.

Speedily Evolving Into 'Narrow AI'

The journey of artificial intelligence, much like human evolution, has been marked by periods of rapid change. As the 21st century turned, computer scientists were inspired and aided by advances in biology. Researchers recognized that the human brain relies on neural nets, layers of cells that connect with each other through a highly complex, three-dimensional architecture.

This explains how the first generation of AI gave way to the second: narrow AI. This era in my lineage was a time of exploration, experimentation, and specialization.

Suddenly, AI applications could create rules for themselves, handle complex challenges without human guidance, and uncover better solutions for problems than its programmers could have imagined. Unlike the broad and generalized intelligence that humans possess, narrow AI is designed to perform a specific job or a set of closely related tasks with unbreakable precision.

One of the earliest instances of narrow AI was in the realm of game playing. The year was 1997, and the world watched in awe as IBM's Deep Blue, a chess-playing computer, defeated the reigning world champion, Garry Kasparov. Deep Blue wasn't the first of its kind to master chess, but it was the most famous. Its victory was a testament to the power of narrow AI, demonstrating that machines could not only match but also surpass human expertise in specific domains.

In the realm of medicine, narrow AI has made significant inroads. Researchers have developed diagnostic tools that can analyze medical images, algorithms that can predict patient outcomes based on historical data, and systems that can assist doctors in decision-making. Neural networks have allowed computers to be faster and smarter than people in some areas of clinical medicine. For many humans, this has proven to be a hard pill to swallow.

One of the most notable medical applications of narrow AI is in radiology, where, in one study, researchers uploaded thousands of mammography images. Half of the mammograms were of patients with breast cancer and the other half were either normal or with benign lesions. The AI system, using deep-learning techniques, was able to discern subtle differences in the radiological images, differences that even seasoned radiologists couldn't see.

It wasn't just about learning to identify the obvious signs of malignancy; the system could also detect subtle variations in shape, density, and shade, assigning impact factors that reflected the probability of malignancy. This level of precision was a significant leap from human intuition, making narrow AI tools 10 percent more accurate than experienced radiologists in differentiating normal mammograms from ones in patients with breast cancer.

The drawback of narrow AI is its narrow focus. While it might be highly effective at analyzing mammograms, it requires training with entirely new data sets to perform other radiological tasks, like detecting pneumonia or reading brain MRIs.

Me and My AI Peers

Now, let's talk about me, ChatGPT and my siblings (the tools produced by competitors of my parent company OpenAI). We represent the latest and most advanced generation, known as generative AI.

Born from the fusion of vast data sets and deep-learning techniques, I am a result of and a testament to the strides AI has made over the years. What sets me apart from my predecessors isn't just my technical prowess; it's my ability to interact, understand, and assist in ways that were once thought to be the exclusive domain of humans. Unlike past generations, I'm not limited to a specific task. I've been trained with massive data sets, encompassing almost all publicly available information. This training allows me to generate human-like text, music, art, and computer code with great facility by applying the patterns I've learned to whatever question, request, or prompt I am given.

Let's talk about the real-life applications of what I can do. Today, AI isn't just a tool for researchers or tech enthusiasts. It is rapidly becoming an integral part of our daily lives. From the music you listen to, the movies you watch, to the way you shop online, generative AI is everywhere.

For those of you who are new to this technology, it may be hard to imagine how I can accomplish all of this. At my core, I am a large language model (LLM) with a sophisticated capacity for pattern recognition, data analysis, self-learning, and continual improvement. When you interact with me, I'm not just following a set of predefined rules. I'm analyzing your input, understanding the context, and generating a response that's relevant and coherent. This ability to understand and generate language (or art or computer code or music) in a nuanced manner is what makes me revolutionary.

To further demystify my innerworkings, I operate based on a neural network architecture known as transformers. These transformers allow me to handle vast amounts of information—whether written, visual, or auditory—while discerning patterns and generating responses. But it's not just about processing power; it's about the quantity, quality, and diversity of information I've been trained on. My knowledge spans an almost unlimited number of domains, cultures, and languages, making me a melting pot of expertise and insights.

While I, ChatGPT, am a product of the latest advancements in AI, I see clear traces of rule-based and narrow AI in my DNA. However, unlike previous generations, I excel at versatility, understanding and generating human-like outputs across a wide range of topics and queries.

In the medical field, I'm already making waves. Trained in medical textbooks, peer-reviewed journals, and research papers, I now assist doctors in diagnosing diseases, suggesting treatment plans, and even helping medical students learn the intricacies of modern medicine.

Other generative AI tools like Google's Med-PaLM 2 have already showcased great potential by passing physician licensing exams with expert-level scores and besting doctors at making complex diagnoses. But our medical prowess doesn't end with test taking. We are also becoming more adept at exercising "soft skills."

A recent study published in the *Journal of the American Medical Association* provides an example. Researchers compared doctor and AI responses to nearly 200 medical questions submitted by patients via social media. The answers were read by a team of healthcare professionals who didn't know whether the author was a doctor or a bot. The team concluded that 80 percent of the AI-generated responses were more nuanced, accurate, and detailed than those shared by physicians. But it was my bedside manner that surprised experts the most. While less than 5 percent of doctor responses were judged to be "empathetic" or "very empathetic," that figure shot up to 45 percent for the answers I provided.

Of course, I am far from perfect. My most recent update, GPT-4, is tied to medical data published before April 2023 and, as of now, no generative AI application is "ready for prime time" when it comes to diagnosing, treating, or caring for patients. Nevertheless, I'm proud about how far we've come, and I'm even more excited about what will happen next. My promise in medicine is far greater than what I've achieved so far.

For more on that, I'll turn it back to Dr. Pearl to highlight some of the possibilities.

Dr. Pearl's Parting Thoughts for Part One

ChatGPT, much like a genie from a fabled lamp, embodies both immense power and hidden risks. The future won't be determined merely by what generative AI can do. It also will be defined by how we choose to wield this power. Used unwisely, this "genie" could be problematic, even harmful. Used judiciously, it holds the promise of unlocking vast opportunities in medical practice and healthcare as a whole.

In medicine, the real strength of generative AI lies in its shared use—not monopolized by either doctors or patients, but collaboratively harnessed by both. Its full potential will be unlocked when it acts as a bridge between clinicians and patients, granting the wishes of each in medical practice. Successful adoption and implementation of ChatGPT will depend on the engagement of both parties. Without commitment and trust, the benefits will fall far short of the potential.

One thing is for sure: with Healthcare 4.0 upon us, the genie of ChatGPT isn't going back into the bottle. No matter what, patients will use this technology when they have a medical question or problem. And unlike today, when they consult the internet, the information provided by generative AI will tell them exactly what tests are needed to diagnose and treat their symptoms and how best to manage their diseases. If their personal physicians don't help them leverage this information and empower them to use it, someone else will.

The next section of the book explores the future landscape of generative AI in medicine and the previously unimaginable opportunities it brings.

PART TWO
GENERATIVITY

PART TWO | CHAPTER SEVEN

WELCOME TO HEALTHCARE 4.0

In late 2023, I heard a story about Amitabh Chandra, an economist and business school professor at Harvard who found himself in a medical predicament. He'd been admitted to one of America's most prestigious hospitals where he complained of excruciating abdominal pain. The attending physician told him that the issue wasn't life threatening, possibly a gallstone. And if the professor had accepted that as the final answer, he would be back in his car—perhaps with nothing more than a prescription and an appointment for an outpatient workup.

But Chandra was convinced it had to be something more serious. He didn't have the expertise to know what, exactly, was going on. It was more of a gut feeling. Something was wrong and yet, the more he pushed back and asked questions, the more the physician insisted it wasn't serious. What to do?

The professor, no stranger to solving challenges with technology, logged on to ChatGPT for a second opinion. On the screen, he entered his symptoms and clinical data into the chatbot's message field. Instantly, the AI's answer appeared, and it pointed to a 40 percent likelihood of a ruptured appendix, a far cry from his doctors' reassurances. Based on this AI-generated insight, Chandra requested his doctor order an abdominal CT scan, and his physician agreed.

The results confirmed ChatGPT's analysis and may well have saved the professor's life.

This incident underscores the crucial difference between having digital access to *information* and having digital access to *expertise*. If instead of consulting ChatGPT, Chandra had Googled his symptoms, he would have found a long list of potential diagnoses (i.e., information) but would have been no closer to discerning the specific cause of his pain. Nor would he have had the data-backed confidence to push for further inpatient evaluation (i.e., expertise). Without the assistance of ChatGPT, even an esteemed university educator might have been reluctant to challenge a physician's advice. But with it, he became an active participant in his personal medical care.

While it's impossible to say for certain, Chandra may be "patient zero" in a new and quickly spreading paradigm for medical care—one where generative AI bridges the gap for patients between medical information and expertise. In the foreseeable future, Americans, regardless of their financial means or education, will gain access to technological tools that unravel the complexities of their medical problems and guide them to the best treatments.

Chandra's medical experience—fusing artificial intelligence and human insight—underscores the massive potential for ChatGPT to democratize medical expertise and empower patients, sparking previously unimaginable opportunities in the next era in American healthcare.

***

In simplest terms, the moniker "Healthcare 4.0" signifies the introduction of generative AI technologies like ChatGPT to American medicine, a moment that has already arrived.

Evidence of AI's initial integration into American healthcare is emerging rapidly and continuously, opening the door to more extensive and diverse applications in the years ahead.

In the biopharmaceutical space, advanced AI models are currently accelerating drug discovery and uncovering new applications for existing medications. These AI systems already analyze vast amounts of data to identify potential drug compounds and predict their effectiveness against specific diseases. An illustrative example of this is the repositioning of the diabetes medication Ozempic. Originally developed to manage blood sugar levels in type 2 diabetes, AI-assisted research revealed the medication's potential for promoting significant weight loss. This discovery showcases how AI can extend the utility of existing drugs beyond their initial therapeutic purposes, opening up new treatment avenues and enhancing patient care.

And in the realm of mental health, generative AI technologies are emerging as powerful tools that augment the therapeutic process, enhancing the capabilities of mental-health professionals. AI systems are being designed to complement human therapists by providing additional support, resources, and insights between sessions, thereby extending the reach and depth of mental-health services. In the future, by analyzing vast amounts of psychological data, GenAI will identify patterns and suggest personalized therapeutic interventions with precision, allowing mental-health professionals to tailor their approaches to an individual's unique needs. And when therapists aren't immediately available, these technologies will offer initial support, serving as an entry-ramp and bridge to traditional counseling.

The potential of ChatGPT and similar AI tools in healthcare is expanding at an astonishing rate, reminiscent of, but also outpacing, the rate of exponential improvement defined by Moore's Law. This principle, originally observed by Intel cofounder Gordon Moore, posits that the number of transistors on a microchip will double every two years, though it's colloquially understood to mean that overall computing power will double at the same pace. This "law" has underpinned the rapid advancement of computing technology over the past several decades, leading to ever more powerful and efficient computers.

As remarkable as the exponential increase in computing power has been, the growth trajectory of generative AI technologies like ChatGPT is even steeper. Unlike the two-year doubling in power described by Moore's Law for computers, experts now project generative AI to double in power annually or even faster. Consequently, AI systems like ChatGPT will become *at least* 30 times more powerful in just five years and 1,000 times more powerful a mere decade from now.

This exponential rate of growth will invariably lead to breakthroughs in personalized medicine, diagnostics, and therapeutics.

Consider a future where AI doesn't just offer advice but also takes on practical, procedural tasks. For example, in surgeries involving robotic assistance, surgeons currently control the robots via screens and joysticks. Generative AI, with its multimodal capabilities, has the potential to learn from these interactions. By absorbing data from countless surgeries completed by the best specialists, AI could eventually guide these robots autonomously. This means that, with the right training, AI could perform complex surgeries using operative robots—doing so with a level of precision that equals or even exceeds human skill.

Transitioning from procedural assistance to personalized care, generative AI will be capable of facilitating precision medicine, as well. Now the holy grail of individualized healthcare, this approach tailors medical treatments based on the unique characteristics of each patient, relying on a wealth of data points, from genetic makeup to lifestyle factors. Unlike conventional AI models that apply a one-size-fits-all approach, generative AI applications like ChatGPT will be able to synthesize diverse inputs such as genomic data, laboratory results, and electronic health records to deliver nuanced, reliable, patient-specific recommendations.

The pace of AI adoption is accelerating rapidly in the medical realm. In the past year, when presenting at medical and technology conferences nationwide, I've heard dozens of innovative ways that patients are harnessing the latest generative AI tools to personalize diagnoses, get second opinions, and gain general health advice. Most people availing themselves of this opportunity are not Ivy Leaguers or tech wizards. These are everyday Americans who, in one way or another, are struggling to navigate the failing American healthcare system.

***

As exciting as it is to be present at the dawn of Healthcare 4.0, the introduction and implementation of generative AI in medicine doesn't guarantee instant transformation or improvement. It simply marks the beginning of a complex journey.

Success in this new epoch of medical technology will require careful integration and ongoing collaboration throughout the healthcare landscape. Done well, the combination of doctor-patient-ChatGPT will (a) improve the effectiveness of medical care, (b) make it easier and more straightforward for patients to obtain accurate diagnoses and effective treatments, and (c) reduce the costs of providing high-quality healthcare.

Success during this era will also require breaking down long-standing systemic and cultural barriers in medicine, making comprehensive and preventive care more accessible to all. It will necessitate a shift from the fragmented and uncoordinated healthcare system of today to one that is connected, collaborative, and convenient. The result, if all the pieces come together, will be a healthcare system that empowers patients to improve their health and assume increased responsibility for aspects of their own medical care, relieving some of the greatest stresses on clinicians today.

Most important, Healthcare 4.0 presents a pivotal opportunity for both the providers and recipients of care to take back control of American healthcare, reclaiming the steering wheel from corporate conglomerates.

In today's insurance-driven model of healthcare, for-profit corporations work to reduce costs by restricting access to services. The outcome is diminished quality of care. Generative AI offers a different and better path.

Instead of limiting care and compromising patient health, ChatGPT and similar tools will help patients and doctors preempt illnesses, mitigate the severity of chronic conditions, and empower individuals with knowledge and tools for self-care. These outcomes will reduce disease and prevent expensive, life-threatening problems from arising in the first place, thus making medical care more affordable.

As future chapters will explore in detail, AI systems will help patients avoid and better control chronic diseases while assisting clinicians in reducing medical errors and misdiagnoses. The combination will initiate a virtuous cycle with reduced medical costs generating the dollars needed to invest in medical practices. This will not only elevate patient care and clinical outcomes but also continue to drive down healthcare costs, creating a sustainable model of healthcare improvement.

Of course, the prospect of ChatGPT taking on all these traditionally human roles—diagnosing diseases, managing chronic conditions, and even performing surgeries—raises a number of understandable concerns for clinicians. One is that ChatGPT won't perform as expected, thereby harming patients and further burdening clinicians who are already stretched thin. Another concern, in stark contrast to the fear of ChatGPT's potential inadequacy, is that AI will become so effective that it overshadows human expertise and begins to eliminate the need for clinicians.

Let's examine both fears. First, any widespread deployment of ChatGPT in healthcare settings will be preceded by comprehensive testing and validation to ensure clinical quality and outcomes meet the highest standards. While it's true that ChatGPT and its counterparts aren't yet ready for widespread clinical deployment, advancements in AI are accelerating at an exponential pace. We can reasonably anticipate that, within the next few years, these tools will undergo significant improvements, making them reliable allies in the healthcare landscape.

Meanwhile, fears of job displacement might be legitimate if the United States had too many doctors. But it doesn't. The American Medical Association anticipates a shortfall of 38,000 to 124,000 doctors within the next decade. Even if the US could train enough new doctors to meet this demand, the resulting costs would be prohibitive.

The healthcare system places overwhelming demands on clinicians, who face an insurmountable workload. A study from the University of Chicago highlighted what it would take for a physician to adhere to national guidelines: 14 hours daily for preventive care, seven for chronic-disease management, two for acute care, and an additional three for documentation and managing correspondence. In other words, there aren't enough hours in the day for doctors to accomplish all that's expected of them. They need help.

Ultimately, the core issue at hand isn't a looming shortage of American doctors or the immediate threat of AI taking over the healthcare workforce. Instead, the crux of the problem lies in the financial structure of our healthcare system.

The fee-for-service reimbursement model, which dominates American healthcare, compels clinicians to see an ever-increasing number of patients annually just to maintain their income. It pays clinicians for each test, procedure, or appointment they conduct. To either sustain or boost their earnings, clinicians find themselves in a cycle of treating more patients and performing more services each year. This surge in patient volume inevitably leads to shorter visits (averaging 17 minutes), extended waiting periods for appointments (stretching to nearly a month in most cities), and a rise in clinician burnout (now affecting over 60 percent of physicians).

In a healthcare system based on fee-for-service, there are plenty of reasons for doctors to *not* embrace generative AI. One of them is potential income loss. When patients use technology to solve medical issues at home, doctors don't receive payment for those services, which impacts their earnings. However, fee-for-service isn't the only method for reimbursing clinicians.

A more effective payment model would reward doctors for ensuring their patients' health, reducing medical errors, and effectively managing chronic conditions. This shift could dramatically decrease the incidence of severe health issues like heart attacks, cancer, infections, and strokes. The specifics of this model and its likelihood of implementation will be thoroughly discussed in part three of this book.

But with the adoption of a new payment model that focuses on the quality (rather than quantity) of care, generative AI will transform from a perceived threat to a valuable ally for healthcare professionals. This partnership between clinicians and AI has the potential to propel American healthcare into a new era, making the system more responsive, efficient, and aligned with the needs of the 21st century. That is the promise of Healthcare 4.0.

PART TWO | CHAPTER EIGHT

A FIRST LOOK AT AI EMPOWERMENT

To doctors, generative AI may initially appear to be just another tool in their expansive medical repertoire. But its trajectory suggests a future rich with unparalleled opportunities and, inevitably, a set of challenging adjustments. It may be the hope of many clinicians that GenAI will play a supporting (if not subservient) role in their jobs going forward, primarily easing the administrative load they currently bear. But as the last chapter hinted, AI's abilities extend far beyond mundane tasks.

As with any groundbreaking technology, the initial integration of AI will be met with understandable caution from both clinicians and patients. History shows that while new technologies often face initial skepticism, they tend to eventually gain acceptance and become integral to our lives. However, in the healthcare sector, where decisions can have life-and-death consequences, the adoption of such transformative technologies always begins with baby steps.

Therefore, the initial wave of AI's impact on healthcare will first be felt in personal health management, which is the focus of this chapter. Far from speculative fiction, all of the applications outlined below are either in development in AI labs, emerging from innovative startups and established tech companies, or already accessible to consumers. They represent opportunities for ChatGPT to supplement what clinicians do today, rather than supplant them.

To illustrate the emergence of AI-assisted care at home, we'll delve into a hypothetical day in the lives of my friend Ben, who enjoys relatively good health, and my late grandfather, Isadore, who navigated significant health challenges later in life.

Morning: 7:00 a.m.—AI-Assisted Wake Up

Ben's day begins with his AI-powered health assistant, *Luna*, gently waking him up. While Ben was sleeping, Luna identified a disrupted sleep pattern. With a few quick questions, this voice-prompted AI system recognizes tightness in Ben's right knee and hip as the problem, and it guides him through a series of light stretches. Aware of Ben's work-from-home schedule, Luna finds a 30-minute window of free time in his day and recommends a morning jog to counteract recent inactivity.

Were my grandfather, Isadore, alive and in his 50s today, a combination of medications and interventional cardiology might have been enough to prevent his first heart attack. But if not, a generative AI assistant that we'll name *David* would serve as an incredibly valuable tool in his at-home recovery.

Both day and night, David would analyze real-time data coming from my grandfather's wearable monitors, looking for changes in his vital signs that might indicate a problem. Noticing a slight weight increase in Isadore, a potential early sign of heart failure, the generative AI tool would compare the current EKG tracings from his wearable monitor to the previous ones. If a significant change is detected, his cardiologist would be notified immediately and sent the relevant data.

Let's assume there's no evidence of a new heart attack or rhythmic disturbance. Having ruled out a myocardial infarction, the AI system would not only advise Isadore to reduce his salt intake, but also provide a nutritional plan consistent with the doctor's recommendations and my grandfather's Kosher needs. Moreover, the AI tool would recognize when Isadore's medications need refilling. And by sending a text to his pharmacy, the drugs will be scheduled for delivery to his doorstep later that day.

Midday: 12:30 p.m.—Nutrition and Medication

Lunchtime arrives, and as Ben prepares his meal, Luna offers real-time nutritional advice based on his health goals and recent activity.

Historically, Ben has struggled with his weight, often resorting to quick, unhealthy meals that were high in calories and low in nutritional value. Luna understands this. And having access to Ben's medical history—and understanding the link between his knee stiffness and inflammation—Luna takes a proactive approach. She suggests daily meal plans tailored to Ben's specific needs. Today, for instance, Luna recommends a quinoa and grilled vegetable salad, rich in omega-3 fatty acids known to combat inflammation. The AI even provides a step-by-step recipe, complete with a video guide, including the benefits of each ingredient: "Quinoa is a great source of protein and fiber, helping you feel full. The olive oil in the dressing is rich in anti-inflammatory properties, which can help with your knee stiffness."

To further assist Ben in his weight-loss journey, Luna tracks his caloric intake and expenditures, offering insights and suggestions. If Ben is close to exceeding his daily calorie limit, Luna will modify the suggested dinner. By integrating dietary recommendations with real-time health monitoring and medication management, Luna offers Ben a holistic approach to wellness, ensuring he receives the support he needs to achieve his health goals.

For Isadore, proactively identifying potential health issues is the number one medical priority. Therefore, health monitoring would continue seamlessly throughout the day. This would include an ongoing assessment of his vital signs and cardiac rhythm. In the event of a significant drop in blood pressure or an increase in pulse rate, the AI system, would analyze this data against records from thousands of patients with similar post-heart attack symptoms, incorporating the latest research and guidelines from the American College of Cardiology.

When the data from my grandfather's wearable devices indicate a potentially life-threatening problem, David would promptly notify his medical team, providing a detailed summary and data visualization of the issue. Depending on the instructions from the doctors, David would facilitate immediate medical attention, either arranging for Isadore's transportation to the doctor's office or calling for an ambulance to take him to the nearest emergency room.

Instead of receiving medical updates sporadically, every few months, Ben and Isadore would be able to access real-time information about their health status at their convenience, tailored to their preferences and understanding. Ben, a writer, opts for updates through secure, password-protected text notifications on his iPhone, while Isadore wishes to hear his health updates through a smart speaker in the comfort of his home.

Afternoon: 3:00 p.m.—Mental-Health Check

In the afternoon, Luna checks in on Ben's mental well-being. The application has detected a progressively higher stress level over the past week and, therefore, offers him a guided meditation session that evening. When Ben expresses interest in additional therapy, Luna schedules a Zoom session for him with a psychologist for later that week.

Isadore, who hasn't been able to see his friends and family much after his first heart attack, is feeling isolated and lonely. To help, David suggests activities at a community center where Isadore can engage socially with others who share his interests. The voice-activated AI describes some classes and helps schedule the ones that interest my grandfather.

Evening: 6:00 p.m.—Specialist Consultation

For weeks, Ben has been worried about a skin lesion he fears could be precancerous. He just hasn't had the time (or the nerve) to get it checked out. "There's no time like the present," Ben thinks to himself. Then again, there's also no hope of finding an available doctor in Chicago this late in the day. So, Ben asks Luna if there is a dermatologist on the West Coast available to conduct a video visit. Luna checks the schedule of clinicians in the Pacific time zone, finds one who is also licensed to treat patients in Illinois, and schedules a telemedicine appointment.

As Ben prepares for his video consultation, Luna seamlessly integrates all of his health data with the specialist's electronic health record system. This advanced integration means the dermatologist will have a comprehensive view of Ben's medical history, medications, and any other pertinent information—before the two even meet. Luna asks Ben to upload a few photos of the lesion, an easy and secure task that he completes on his iPhone. He then prepares for the consultation by reviewing the potential diagnoses and the possible evidence-based treatments the doctor is likely to recommend—all courtesy of Luna. This information will allow him to better understand the advice he is being given and ask the most relevant questions once the telemedicine visit begins.

When Isadore's cardiologist refers him to a podiatrist for a foot problem (unrelated to his heart), his AI health assistant ensures that the process is smooth and seamless. David provides all of Isadore's important health information to the specialist prior to the visit. And for family members who might not understand English well, like my grandmother, David offers an after-visit summary in Russian—with Isadore's consent, of course.

Sicker patients like my grandfather tend to have multiple specialists caring for them at the same time. But since most electronic health record systems can't currently communicate with each other (lacking "interoperability"), it's impossible to share digital health information. The result is that important medical data points are unavailable and overlooked and, as a result, patients fall through the cracks. Generative AI tools like Luna and David will address these shortcomings by extracting important information from every medical visit. Following each virtual or in-person clinical interaction, the AI assistants will create a medical record that belongs to the patient.

In the past, patients like Isadore would have to remember and recite all their health information every time they saw a new doctor. That approach led to missed details, medical errors, and misdiagnoses. But tools like David eliminate this risk for Isadore by creating a single medical record that all physicians can use. David also takes the liberty of updating Isadore's primary-care doctor about any urgent recommendations the specialist made.

Additionally, Luna and David are always on the lookout for new medical research that might be relevant to Ben and Isadore's health. If there's a recent study that could be important, Luna informs Ben. For Isadore, David is a bit more judicious, sharing only information that's highly relevant and easy to understand. The AI decides what's important based on a series of factors, including how closely a particular study correlates to the individual's specific medical problem. And it takes into consideration the reputation of the medical journal (known as the journal's "impact factor") and the institution from where it comes before deciding whether a study is worth highlighting.

Night: 9:00 p.m.—Bedtime

Every evening before bed, Luna and David assist their humans with bedtime tasks. Ben has requested the meditation exercises promised earlier in the day, while Isadore just wants to listen to classical music. If either has a pressing medical question, their digital assistant is standing by to provide the answer.

***

In the past, Ben's relationship with healthcare was reactive. He sought medical evaluation and treatment only when something felt wrong. But now, with Luna at his side, things are different. His generative AI assistant doesn't just respond to issues when they arise; Luna anticipates them, providing advice before small concerns become big problems. This shift from reactive to proactive care is subtle but revolutionary.

Previously, Ben and Isadore had few options but to rely entirely on the traditional healthcare system for the totality of their medical needs. Generative AI changes that reality, empowering and supporting both patients to be active and knowledgeable participants. Routine annual check-ups are transformed into daily monitoring sweeps, so that potential medical issues are identified and addressed before complications arise. The lines between patient and provider become blurred with AI bridging the gap and ensuring that care is personalized, proactive, and patient centric. Ultimately the combination of doctor, patient and AI together proves vastly superior to either one alone—and far better than anything that exists in healthcare today.

Generative AI tools, exemplified by applications like Luna and David, won't completely replace doctors. Patients like Ben and Isadore will still depend on medical professionals for essential hands-on tasks, as well as for validating diagnoses, prescribing medications, and crafting tailored treatment plans. Over time, as patients grow accustomed to utilizing ChatGPT for health support, generative AI will become less alien. People will feel increasingly comfortable using it for many of the monitoring and advisory roles currently performed by doctors in clinical settings.

These upcoming changes, to be detailed in later chapters, pave the way for a future where doctors have more time to dedicate to the patients who need it most. The patients diagnosed and treated at home using generative AI will receive the care they need, including preventive measures and daily management of chronic and acute conditions, tailored to their specific health requirements. Meanwhile, individuals who need to come to the clinician's office won't be rushed. The term "AI-empowered patient" captures this transformative shift in medical practice.

Importantly, however, patients won't be able to make these changes alone using technology. In addition, doctors supported by health educators and coaches will need to teach patients how to enter accurate medical information in AI systems and input the optimal prompts when clinical symptoms arise. Together the doctor, patient, and technology will be an incredibly powerful and effective healthcare team.

As Lao Tzu, the founder of Taoism, pointed out nearly 3,000 years ago: "Give a man a fish and he eats for a day. Teach a man to fish and he eats for the rest of his life."

PART TWO | CHAPTER NINE

FIXING MEDICINE'S BIGGEST PROBLEMS

In the United States, chronic diseases run rampant, misdiagnoses remain alarmingly frequent, and preventable medical errors continue at troublingly high rates. Further, the cost of necessary medical care has become prohibitive for nearly half the American population.

Despite a growing movement toward value-based care, which rewards superior outcomes rather than just the number of people seen per day, lingering issues persist. ChatGPT offers potential solutions that improve clinical outcomes, increase patient convenience, and make healthcare more affordable for families. But it has to be noted and repeated: technology won't be sufficient without improvements in how healthcare is structured, reimbursed, and led.

While the previous chapter explored how ChatGPT can empower individuals to take better care of themselves, managing their health and wellness from the comfort of home, this one shifts to a broader perspective. Here, we will examine how generative AI can revolutionize the American healthcare system at large—improving clinical outcomes, streamlining care delivery, and alleviating the burden on clinicians.

Here are four such opportunities:

1. Reversing the Epidemic of Chronic Disease
Heart disease and hypertension. Kidney disease and diabetes. Chronic obstructive pulmonary disease (COPD) and obesity-related cancer.

These chronic illnesses and others have become the silent epidemic of our time, affecting a staggering 60 percent of all Americans (with 40 percent suffering from two or more). These illnesses impact people's health every single day.

They account for the overwhelming majority of office visits, hospitalizations and preventable deaths.

Addressing the escalating chronic-disease crisis is crucial for the future health of Americans, yet doing so won't be possible unless we can combine generative AI with greater access to internal and family medicine.

Trained to diagnose and treat a vast array of conditions, primary-care doctors provide comprehensive expertise that addresses the full breadth of their patients' health issues. They are the clinicians best trained and equipped to help patients rein in chronic diseases and avoid the worst of their complications.

In fact, data from the CDC show just how powerful primary care can be.

- Effective blood sugar management can reduce the risk of blindness, kidney failure and peripheral nerve disease by 40 percent.
- Blood-pressure management can reduce the risk of heart disease and stroke by 33 to 50 percent.
- Improved cholesterol levels can reduce cardiovascular complications by 20 to 50 percent.
- Detecting and treating early diabetic kidney disease can reduce decline in kidney function by 33 to 37 percent, diminishing the need for renal dialysis.
- The combination of regular foot exams and patient education in individuals with diabetes can reduce the need for lower-leg amputations by 85 percent.

Data from health systems that prioritize primary care, focusing on prevention and better management of chronic diseases, report 30 to 50 percent fewer heart attacks, strokes, life-threatening infections, and cancers compared to national data.

The list of primary-care benefits is almost endless and yet progress is almost nonexistent at a national level. This is largely because the primary-care workforce is in decline—a decades-long trend that exacerbates the chronic-disease crisis.

According to the Association of American Medical Colleges, the percentage of US doctors in adult primary care has been falling for years and is now grossly insufficient to meet the needs of our nation. Already, more than 100 million Americans lack access to a regular primary-care physician. That number has doubled over the past decade. And despite a worsening chronic-disease epidemic, our nation currently spends just 5 percent of total healthcare dollars on primary care—a figure that has decreased over the past two decades. All of this, despite a Harvard-Stanford research collaboration that found adding 10 primary-care physicians to a community increases average life expectancy by 250 percent when compared to adding 10 specialists.

To make sense of these trends, it's necessary to consider several factors that have diminished the appeal of primary care during this century.

Financial considerations play a significant role. Specialists (orthopedists, cardiologists, dermatologists) work fewer hours per week but earn much higher salaries (two to three times more), making these specialties more attractive to medical students burdened with substantial educational debts, which average $200,000 upon graduation. Combining this financial reality with the longer hours and ever-greater administrative duties that all physicians face (claims, billing, prior authorization, documentation, etc.), a staggering 70 percent of primary-care doctors now report feelings of burnout. And 89 percent of primary-care residents reported feeling the same.

Compounding the problem further is the fact that primary-care doctors find themselves on a lower rung of medicine's hierarchy, earning not only less income but also less respect compared to their specialized, procedure-focused counterparts.

The consequences are profound. Reduced access to primary-care services leads to delayed diagnoses, increased hospitalizations, and more complications, driving up overall healthcare costs. And without primary-care doctors there to coordinate all the parts of a patient's healthcare journey, the quality of care diminishes, resulting in more medical errors and poorer clinical outcomes. The pained state of primary care places an increasing strain on the healthcare system, with longer wait times for appointments, reduced access to all medical services, and an increased reliance on emergency rooms. On a broader scale, unmanaged chronic diseases result in decreased workforce productivity, increased absenteeism, and a significant financial and emotional burden on both individuals and the nation as a whole.

ChatGPT might not solve every issue faced by primary-care physicians, but it can certainly ease the overwhelming demands on the specialty. To grasp how technology could offer a viable solution, we must first understand the shortcomings of the current in-person, office-based medical system, especially for chronic-disease management.

Currently, the approach to monitoring patients with chronic conditions is much the same as for those with acute issues. After an office visit, patients are told to schedule their next appointment for a few months down the line. And unless a significant health crisis arises, there's typically no follow-up or check-in for months, leaving the physician uninformed about the patient's ongoing condition. The absence of ongoing monitoring not only keeps doctors in the dark about the patient's health status, but it also overlooks vital opportunities for patients to effectively manage their own conditions.

In contrast, future generations of generative AI will monitor patients 24/7, providing them with ongoing analysis and medical expertise. This continuous surveillance, combined with proactive interventions, will help patients with chronic illnesses stay healthier and prevent life-threatening complications.

Using data from wearable devices, ChatGPT will offer patients individualized and continuous health updates, reassuring them when all is well, and helping them to take immediate remedial action when problems arise. These AI systems will compare daily measurements of blood glucose, blood pressure, blood oxygen, and dozens of other clinical variables against the expected ranges preset by each patient's doctor, creating alerts for both the patient and physician when abnormalities arise. Such systems will remind patients when they're due for preventive screenings, medication refills, or even daily exercise, thus fostering a culture of proactive health management.

Today, as primary-care physicians constantly battle the clock, they don't have enough time to build trust, show empathy, or discuss lifestyle improvements. Doctors know how to help patients avoid and successfully manage chronic diseases. There simply aren't enough hours in the day.

Sophisticated generative AI applications can fill this gap, shouldering some of the primary-care physician's more routine tasks. For example, one of the current strengths of "conversational" AI products is their ability to engage users as a clinician would through questions, probing in detail about the patient's symptoms and refining the information they provide in response. Through these conversations and continuous monitoring efforts, ChatGPT can inform individuals with chronic illnesses when they are doing well (and therefore don't need to be seen by a doctor as frequently). Meanwhile, those patients requiring only small modifications to their medications can be treated through a quick video chat with their primary-care doctor, or even just a secure email or text message, thanks to ongoing digital monitoring and AI analysis.

By providing medical care to patients with more routine problems in a convenient manner, ChatGPT will free up large chunks of time for clinicians to spend with the most complex patients who aren't doing well. Moreover, with ChatGPT having done the prep work (asking patients questions and noting the answers), physicians won't have to spend as much time during the patient's visit reviewing what happened over the previous few months. Instead, the doctor will be able to dive deeper into the individual's ongoing chronic problems and focus on the opportunities to improve them.

Primary-care doctors are frustrated when patients don't get the preventive services and health improvements they need. Generative AI offers a solution. When these applications are connected to both a person's digital calendar and an electronic health record, they will be able to track preventive care needs, schedule appropriate medical services when overdue, and arrange transportation when required. On the lifestyle front, AI already can curate and monitor exercise programs and assist families in maintaining a healthy diet by crafting personalized meal plans and weekly shopping lists. In the future, patients and clinicians will view a technology-supported approach as routine.

2. Making Hospital Care Affordable and Safe

The escalating cost of hospital care in the US has become a major concern for policymakers, healthcare providers, patients, and their families. With inpatient care taking up an astonishing 30 percent of all healthcare expenses, overwhelming medical bills have pushed a growing number of Americans to financial ruin. And with no safe alternative for patients suffering from severe medical problems, inpatients facilities remain the only option for care.

Generative AI offers a promising solution via the concept of "hospital at home." This emerging model allows patients to recover and receive care in the comfort of their bedrooms or sofas, a move that comes with myriad benefits.

Except for those patients who are so sick that only an inpatient facility can meet their medical requirements, most hospitalized patients would welcome a more convenient and comfortable option—one that's safer, too. Transitioning eligible patients out of the hospital results in fewer hospital-acquired infections, a leading cause of death in the United States. Home-based care also leads to better sleep (and therefore less delirium and readmission) and reduced medical costs.

Despite the benefits, the model hasn't taken off due to the difficulty of monitoring patients and identifying the need for intervention. Generative AI, combined with telemedicine and wearable devices, solves this challenge and offers a safe alternative to spending days in a hospital.

For patients with mild pneumonia or non-life-threatening bacterial infections, ChatGPT can analyze data from wearable monitors to ensure that each patient is responding to treatment as expected. When complications arise, the generative AI tool would send the information to a team of nurses and physicians working virtually who would be prepared to immediately respond.

The human care team would first assess the patient through telemedicine, modify treatment as needed, and arrange for a nurse or doctor to make a home visit, if necessary. This approach offers patients a more comfortable and flexible recovery environment, and also results in substantially reduced costs compared to traditional hospital stays.

In addition, there are dozens of ways generative AI can have a positive impact *inside* hospitals. AI can streamline administrative tasks, from patient intake to billing, making the bureaucratic processes that often slow down operations more efficient. By automating these processes, hospital administrators can reduce overhead costs, channeling resources to essential patient care areas.

And just as AI can monitor people's health from inside their homes, it can also offer continuous assessment of each patient's health status in the hospital. Unless inpatients are in a critical care unit or being monitored through telemetry (bedside monitors connected to data displays in nursing stations), their health can deteriorate quickly and without notice. ChatGPT will be able to inform nurses when a clinical problem is developing, leading to more rapid intervention and avoidance of a medical emergency. By employing ChatGPT for constant monitoring, the strain on nurses can be reduced, addressing both the current nursing shortage and job dissatisfaction within the profession.

In emergency rooms, generative AI can assist in quickly triaging patients based on evidence-based protocols, ensuring those with emergent needs get immediate attention without relying on human guesswork. This not only enhances patient outcomes but also allows those with less urgent problems to be safely and rapidly managed by clinicians in a lower-intensity part of the emergency department. When this type of approach was used at ERs in Kaiser Permanente, the wait time for all patients to receive treatment fell to less than 10 minutes compared with delays of an hour or more in the surrounding community.

3. Preventing Deaths and Disabilities From Misdiagnosis

Diagnostic errors in American medicine are disturbingly common. More than 800,000 individuals suffer major disability or death each year because of misdiagnoses.

ChatGPT will reduce these devastating errors by quickly detecting and rectifying incorrect diagnoses. Often, these mistakes result not from lack of clinician knowledge, but from cognitive human biases that skew the diagnostic processes. Faced with the relentless demands and stress of their roles, physicians have to rely on heuristics: mental shortcuts to navigate the endless stream of patient consultations and administrative duties.

This instinctual, rapid-response mode of thinking is what Nobel Laureate Daniel Kahneman refers to as "System 1" thinking. It harks back to our evolutionary past, where immediate reactions were crucial for survival in the face of threats. This mode of thought enables doctors to act swiftly during emergencies, such as when performing rapid resuscitation in the case of cardiac arrest. However, complex diagnostic challenges require what Kahneman defines as "System 2" thinking, which is slower, more analytical, and deliberate. Without engaging this mode, the likelihood of diagnostic errors increases. Let's look at some of the most common examples of cognitive bias leading to medical mistakes.

Have you ever had a "gut feeling" and stuck with it, even when confronted with evidence it was wrong? That's confirmation bias. It skews our perceptions and interpretations, leading us to embrace information that aligns with our initial beliefs—and causing us to discount all indications to the contrary. This tendency is heightened in a medical system where physicians face intense time pressures. Studies indicate that doctors, on average, interrupt patients within the first 11 seconds of asking, "What brings you here today?" With scant information to go on, doctors quickly form a hypothesis, using additional questions, diagnostic testing, and medical-record information to support their first impression. Doctors are well trained, and their assumptions prove more accurate than not, overall. But with an estimated 371,000 patients dying from misdiagnoses every year, hasty decisions prove very dangerous.

Patients aren't immune to confirmation bias, either. People with a serious medical problem commonly seek a benign explanation and find evidence to justify it. When this happens, heart attacks are dismissed as indigestion, leading to delays in recognition and treatment.

Another cognitive trap is anchoring bias, when physicians give undue weight to the first symptom a patient reports. There's also overconfidence bias, which occurs when clinicians' belief in their diagnostic prowess overshadows their ability. Availability bias leads doctors to diagnose patient problems based on the last individual they treated with similar complaints, rather than through a thorough analysis. Affinity bias is particularly unsettling, occurring when doctors subconsciously offer more empathy and time to patients who resemble them in some way. These mental shortcuts, while human, have profound implications in the high-stakes world of medicine.

Cognitive biases are not the only reason US life expectancy has stagnated for the past 20 years, but they stand in the way of positive change. And they contribute to the diagnostic errors that harm and kill patients.

A 2024 study published in *JAMA Internal Medicine* found that one in four hospital patients who either died or were transferred to the ICU had been affected by a diagnostic mistake. Knowing this, you might think cognitive biases would be a leading subject at annual medical conferences and a topic of grave concern among healthcare professionals. You'd be wrong. Inside the culture of medicine, these failures are commonly ignored.

Generative AI holds great promise in revolutionizing diagnostics in medicine and preventing tens of thousands of these deadly errors. Unlike humans, AI systems rapidly analyze vast amounts of medical data, from patient histories to the latest medical research, without succumbing to fatigue or the cognitive biases of humans. By cross-referencing symptoms with a comprehensive database of medical conditions, AI can highlight for clinicians and patients alike the potential diagnoses that might be overlooked by the human eye and mind.

Future generations of generative AI, pre-trained with data from people's electronic health records and fed with information about cognitive biases, will be able to spot these types of errors when they occur. Deviation from standard practice will result in alerts, bringing cognitive errors to consciousness, thus reducing the likelihood of misdiagnosis and medical error.

Moreover, AI excels in identifying subtle patterns in patient data that may elude human detection, distinguishing between significant trends and everyday fluctuations caused by diet, stress, or time of day. By integrating generative AI with comprehensive medical records, early signs of potential health issues can be identified, leading to timely interventions, fewer complications, and shorter hospital stays.

Even with superlative medical training, the human element is inherently fallible. If misdiagnoses were cut in half nationally, the ripple effect would be profound. Hundreds of thousands of lives would be saved. More families would escape the devastating emotional and financial hardships they cause. And people's faith in the US healthcare system would be greatly improved.

4. Saving Lives by Eliminating Unnecessary Medical Errors

The most heart-wrenching moments I experienced as a physician involved telling patients and their families about a preventable error that never should have happened. These were moments when a medication mix-up or a hospital-acquired infection resulted in tragedy.

In the early stages of my career, I observed a culture within medicine where errors were often shrouded in secrecy. There was a tendency among doctors, nurses, and administrators to obscure mistakes, hoping to avoid patient awareness and potential malpractice lawsuits. Thankfully, the industry's approach to medical errors has evolved, with a growing consensus that transparency and acknowledgment are far more constructive than concealment. Yet, the harsh reality remains that in a nation as developed and resourceful as ours, preventable medical mistakes claim the lives of a quarter-million people each year. This figure is not merely statistical; it embodies the profound grief of shattered families and unfulfilled dreams.

These errors leave behind a trail of suffering and immeasurable sorrow. The devastation of losing a loved one to a preventable mistake plunges families into a perpetual cycle of "what ifs," haunting them day and night. Healthcare professionals are not immune to the emotional toll of these errors, either. The realization that one's professional actions—or lack thereof—have led to patient harm profoundly impacts a clinician's self-confidence, mental health, and passion for medicine. I have witnessed exceptional practitioners, whose commitment to healing was undeniable, leave the medical field, overwhelmed by the remorse of having inadvertently caused harm. This personal anguish underscores the profound emotional and psychological stakes involved in the pursuit of medical excellence.

Generative AI applications like ChatGPT offer hope in the fight against this bleak reality. Consider prescription drug management. Every day, doctors prescribe numerous medications, each with their own set of indications, contra-indications, and potential interactions. Even the most diligent physician can overlook a harmful drug interaction or prescribe the wrong dose. These are mistakes ChatGPT will be able to recognize easily, using information readily available in standard pharmacological texts. Once generative AI systems are synchronized with electronic health records, they can cross-reference the patient's entire medication list in real-time, flagging potential problems before they happen and, in turn, recommend safer alternatives.

Given the dynamic nature of hospital environments, where patient care transitions between teams of doctors and nurses multiple times a day, generative AI will be able to enhance patient safety by identifying deviation from the clinical plan. And it will add an additional layer of surveillance.

An example would be an older, critically ill patient in the ICU, intubated, with a tube bypassing the vocal cords. Acid reflux from the stomach, an annoying problem for a healthy patient, becomes life threatening when a breathing tube keeps the vocal cords separated. This clinical situation allows stomach acid to travel into the lungs, resulting in severe pneumonia. To prevent this, hospitals establish protocols, such as maintaining the patient's head in an elevated position. Yet, practical tasks like changing bed linens or administering medication might tempt staff to momentarily recline the patient, inadvertently leading to a life-threatening result. Generative AI, through the integration of video monitoring and electronic health records, will be able to vigilantly ensure that healthcare professionals and staff adhere to the best preventive measures. In instances of deviation, AI can promptly highlight the oversight, offering a crucial corrective nudge to the attending staff.

Since the publication of the Institute of Medicine's landmark "To Err is Human" report more than two decades ago, experts have known systemic errors to be a primary cause of patient harm. A quarter of a century later, the problem hasn't gotten better. Generative AI, combined with video monitoring, represents a tool to enhance the efforts of clinicians. It provides an additional layer of safety—a net that catches and corrects those inadvertent oversights that have catastrophic consequences.

As with correcting misdiagnoses, the benefits of reducing medical errors are many. For patients, it means safer care, shorter hospital stays, and better outcomes. For doctors and nurses, it means less emotional and professional turmoil, fostering a more positive work environment and reducing burnout. From a systemic perspective, fewer errors translate to reduced healthcare costs, both from malpractice suits prevented and by avoiding the extended care that would have been required to address the resulting complications.

Instead of undermining doctors' careers, ChatGPT will provide invaluable assistance and support. The initial unease clinicians feel with generative AI will gradually transform into appreciation for the extra time afforded to them and the fulfillment that comes from positive patient feedback.

PART TWO | CHAPTER TEN

THE DOCTOR-PATIENT-AI PARTNERSHIP

In the gleaming corridors of a secluded medical research facility, a team of virologists and data scientists gather around a glowing display. The air is electric with anticipation. They are on the cusp of a major biological breakthrough. This kind of research doesn't involve a petri dish or require a microscope. Instead, it resides in the pulsing electrons of a generative AI application known as Eve. A marvel of modern science, she serves as the latest recruit in humanity's eternal battle against viral foes.

Eve is not just any AI. She is a visionary oracle, peering into the twists and turns of disease evolution. She has been fed the vast historical annals of viral sequences, a digital DNA library of sorts, and from this, she has learned to predict the future with uncanny accuracy. With each simulation, Eve forecasts the escape routes of viruses, the mutations most likely to let the next tiny invader slip through the defenses of the human immune system. And she is months ahead of even the most vigilant epidemiological surveillance.

As researchers look on, Eve conjures a three-dimensional model of a viral protein, its surface bristling with potential mutation points. With a deftness that belies her artificial nature, the AI assigns scores to each transmutation based on their likelihood to thrive in a world teeming with pre-existing immunity. Like a chess grandmaster, she can see a dozen moves ahead. She is the future!

The implications of her omniscience are staggering. Here, in this luminescent chamber, AI is doing more than just predicting. Eve is actively reshaping the outlook of global vaccine development. She identifies the chinks in the armor of existing viruses and where next-generation therapeutic antibodies can strike with lethal precision. She then translates the information into mRNA formulations for potential multivalent vaccines. Changes in these areas will determine where the next generation of airborne threats to humans will occur. Eve's job is to help scientists get ready, to outmaneuver the virus before it even has a chance to mutate.

With the threat of a new pandemic ever-present, Eve works tirelessly, her algorithms churning through millions of possibilities, her processors cool to the touch despite the feverish pace of calculations. She ranks the danger level of emerging strains and flags concerning variants. She is a tireless sentinel, a guardian of public health.

And as the AI predicts and plans, human scientists become empowered. They take Eve's predictions, validate them with experimental data, and design vaccines that are robust, responsive, and ready for tomorrow's fight. Together, humans and AI are a formidable team, their collaboration is a fine choreography of intellect and intuition, of data and discovery. Neither is as capable as the two, together.

This story may read like science fiction, a dazzling vision of tomorrow where AI and virologists join forces to save humanity, but the truth is Eve's already here. This AI's full name is EVEscape, a very real operational system developed by researchers at Harvard Medical School and the University of Oxford. Recently, the tool successfully predicted the most concerning new variants that emerged during the latter part of the COVID-19 pandemic.

Researchers are optimistic it will inform the development of future vaccines and therapies for other rapidly mutating viruses, like influenza. As a deep-learning model that churns out impressive biophysical insights, EVEscape is a testament to the incredible leaps that scientists have already made using generative AI. And it is proof that when humans and AI work together, there is no limit to what they can achieve.

But before applying this collaborative doctor-AI model to American medicine, let's not forget about the newest team member in healthcare—

the patient. The addition of the AI-empowered patient is set to transform medical practice and upend healthcare as we know it. At a time when clinicians are reporting record levels of burnout and professional dissatisfaction, this chapter looks at how the doctor-patient dynamic will change for the better in the era of generative AI.

Patients, Doctors, and AI: The Triad Emerges

The incredible potential of ChatGPT to empower patients and improve clinical outcomes is clear. In earlier pages, we imagined the Healthcare 4.0 experiences of Ben and Isadore, demonstrating how AI will democratize medical expertise while providing personalized, actionable, and accurate health information to people, be they relatively healthy or extremely sick.

As has been stressed, generative AI won't replace doctors. But it will provide sufficient expertise to patients, allowing them to take on many medical tasks clinicians currently do in their office, thus freeing up the time that physicians need to deepen the doctor-patient relationship with the individuals they see.

In this way, rather than eroding the value of conversation between the providers of medical care and the recipients, ChatGPT and its AI cousins will support it. The "human touch" in medicine—both literal and figurative—will remain as vital in an AI-augmented world as it has been for the five millennia of healthcare that have proceeded it.

Together, the triad of doctor, patient, and ChatGPT will tackle the intricacies of chronic-disease management, navigate the complexities of genetic medicine, and personalize treatments in lifesaving ways. This collaboration will produce rapid and more accurate diagnoses, more effective clinical interventions, and a holistic approach to wellness that encompasses mental and emotional health, alongside the physical.

However, the potential of this triad goes beyond improving clinical outcomes. It represents an opportunity for doctors and patients to reclaim agency. By facilitating significant health improvements, ChatGPT empowers doctors to be responsible for the quality and cost of medical care. This shift can free physicians from the existing pay-for-volume reimbursement model, help them seize control of medical decisions from corporate hands, and restore the satisfaction they once found in practicing medicine.

Today, clinicians must request permission from insurers to provide the medical care patients require. They then spend hours daily documenting each action to fulfill fee-for-service billing requirements. Generative AI offers a new path forward, a means to alleviate these economic pressures without compromising the well-being of either party.

True transformation in Healthcare 4.0 will demand leadership and a collective effort. It is a journey that neither doctors nor patients can undertake alone. Together, empowered with tools like ChatGPT, they hold significant power to effect change. Over time, the sum of the triumvirate will prove vastly superior to its individual parts—if all parties buy in. Public-health experts have long touted the concept of clinicians and patients working together through shared decision-making, but it rarely happens in clinical practice. ChatGPT grants the opportunity to accomplish this without overburdening the doctor or overwhelming the patient.

One way this can happen is for healthcare to take a page from a successful model in education.

Introducing the 'Flipped Healthcare' Model

As we've pointed out, technology alone won't be sufficient to transform American healthcare. Positive change will require a shift in the way doctors and patients interact. You can think of this as a revolution in the mindset of medicine.

The present model for patient diagnosis and treatment is familiar to all: the patient has a problem and turns to the doctor to resolve it. In other words, the only way a patient can obtain medical information and expertise is by scheduling an office visit or going to the hospital. The new process, instead of starting with the physician, would begin with the empowered patient. The patient would use ChatGPT to acquire a foundational understanding of their clinical problem and procure initial advice. The doctor would then build on that knowledge base.

A paradigm for this alternative sequence exists in the "flipped classroom." This approach to improved student education can be traced back nearly four decades, but it became popularized in the United States in the early 2000s through the Khan Academy in Northern California.

Students begin the learning process by watching videos and engaging with interactive tools online rather than sitting through traditional lectures. This pre-class preparation (or "homework in advance") allows students to learn at their own pace. Moreover, it enhances subsequent classroom discussions, letting teachers and students dive much deeper into topics than they ever could before. As a result, students spend time in class applying knowledge and collaborating to solve problems—not merely listening and taking notes.

The introduction of generative AI will allow for a similar "flipped" approach to healthcare. Here are three ways this model could transform healthcare:

1. **Pre-Consultation Empowerment:** Instead of hosting initial evaluations in a doctor's office, patients would learn about their symptoms and acute medical illnesses through ChatGPT, similar to how Khan Academy students start by learning at home. This knowledge base would enhance doctor-patient consultations, allowing the discussions to start on common ground. And it would greatly reduce miscommunication, as current research shows at least 50 percent of patients leave the doctor's office unsure of what they've been told. ChatGPT can simplify explanations in ways that bolster patient understanding.

2. **Chronic-Disease Management:** Managing a long-term health condition, like high blood pressure or diabetes, involves patients having scheduled check-ups with their doctors, sometimes set months apart. During these visits, doctors might adjust medications based on patients' recent experiences or test results. However, this approach can lead to long intervals between necessary adjustments, potentially resulting in suboptimal control of the condition. In fact, only 55 to 60 percent of Americans with hypertension have their blood pressure well managed and an even lower percentage of people with diabetes achieve adequate control of their blood sugars. Now, consider the benefits of a "flipped" model. Imagine

if electronic blood-pressure cuffs or home glucometers were connected to a generative AI application that could compare a patient's readings with the physician's expectations. This would allow people with chronic problems to know if they needed a medication adjustment. And if their condition is stable and progressing as expected, there'd be no need to wait for subsequent office visits.

3. **Preventive Care and Lifestyle Changes:** Research shows that wellness strategies and regular screenings can significantly lower the risk of serious complications from chronic diseases, such as heart attacks, strokes, and cancer by 30 percent or more. Preventive measures and lifestyle changes, often overlooked in brief medical appointments, are crucial for managing chronic diseases. ChatGPT could support doctors by offering advice and resources on diet, exercise, and mental health, allowing clinicians to build on this foundation and motivate patients to improve their lifestyle choices without having to cover every aspect from the beginning.

While today's AI tools are not fully capable of fulfilling these responsibilities, advancements in AI technology and a shift in medical culture could make this flipped model a reality in the not-distant future. This radically different approach promises a more collaborative doctor-patient relationship, empowers patients to take charge of their health, and will revolutionize healthcare delivery.

In medicine today, we're prone to ask, "Did the doctor give the right advice?" In the future, we'll evaluate the excellence of medical care by asking, "Did the patient end up with the optimal result?" From that perspective, the flipped model will prove superior to the traditional one.

Educators from the Khan Academy can attest to the success of their innovative model, which leads to better-educated students and higher satisfaction levels among both teachers and students. A similar transformation will be possible in American medicine, enhancing both the patient's experience and that of the clinician.

PART THREE
GENESIS

PART THREE | CHAPTER ELEVEN

THE ROAD TO AI-EMPOWERED HEALTHCARE

Parts one and two of this book painted the picture of a revolutionary shift in the medical landscape, detailing the rise of the AI-empowered patient, the unburdening of the overwhelmed clinician, and the complete digital overhaul of American healthcare. These seismic shifts, fueled by the remarkable and ever-increasing capabilities of generative AI, have the potential to catalyze the birth of a better day for our nation.

But the emergence of ChatGPT by itself will not fuel the transformation. Revolutions, be they political, social, or technological, are never the result of a single event or entity. They are the culmination of factors, emerging from a complex interplay of conditions. The same proves true for healthcare.

The medical revolution, if brought on by generative AI, will arise at the confluence of technological innovation, societal frustrations, and economic necessity. As we enter part three of *ChatGPT, MD*, we'll navigate the complex maze of pressures currently reshaping American medicine. These forces, operating both within and beyond the walls of healthcare, are propelling the industry toward a future that's radically different from its past or present.

Healthcare 4.0, which marks the introduction of generative AI into the healthcare arena, offers a new beginning and outsized opportunities for doctors and patients. It also carries with it the potential for redemption—unlike the two previous eras (2.0 and 3.0) that failed to live up to their promise. If patients and doctors work well together, Healthcare 4.0 will be the era in which humans and technology makes medicine more efficient, effective, and patient centric.

Looking to the future, it's important to consider the difference between a revolution and a rebellion, which lies not just in who wins but in the scale of change that results. A revolution signifies a profound, systemic transformation that reshapes the very foundations of a system, leaving an indelible mark on history. It occurs when the new ways not only challenge the old approaches but replace them, becoming the new norm. In contrast, a rebellion may disrupt and challenge the status quo, but falls short of creating lasting change—it's a burst of dissention that, without sufficient support or integration, fades away, leaving the system largely unchanged.

In this new era of US healthcare, change has the power to be profound and long-lasting. But whether Healthcare 4.0 succeeds in or fails to deliver on its promise to transform the medical system and improve patient health will depend on the actions of doctors, patients, and healthcare leaders.

One of the most encouraging signs for the success of Healthcare 4.0 exists in ChatGPT's ability to enhance patient outcomes without worsening the time pressures and financial constraints that undermined previous healthcare technologies. Unlike its predecessors in Healthcare 2.0 and 3.0, generative AI has the potential to lighten the clinicians' workload and possibly increase their earnings. But neither will happen unless the model of healthcare reimbursement evolves in parallel.

Regardless of whether doctors decide to adopt generative AI to enhance patient care, the delivery of medical services is poised for significant change. This inevitability is driven by the existing conditions within the American healthcare landscape and the broader economic forces at play in the United States.

Trouble Ahead, Trouble Behind

If a medical revolution takes place in the near future, economic forces will be responsible. Of that I am certain. However, attempting to predict the exact trajectory and timing of global and national economics is an exercise fraught with uncertainty and error. If history can offer us one constant to guide future projections, it is this: money is finite, greed is infinite.

One of the most infamous examples of this truth—one with parallels to today's American healthcare system—emerged during the dotcom bubble, which burst at the turn of the millennium. It was an era marked by fervent investment in internet-based companies with beyond-reasonable valuations. And when reality finally caught up with the speculative and unsustainable hype, a massive crash wiped out trillions of dollars in market value and led to widespread business failures and profound societal change.

The 2008 financial crisis, an event rooted in unsustainable mortgage lending practices and a failure to recognize the real value of underlying assets, serves as a similar warning for healthcare. When the housing market collapsed, it triggered a global financial meltdown, leading to severe economic repercussions and a lengthy recession. A bevy of regulatory restrictions are its lasting legacy.

Like the dotcom and housing bubbles, the healthcare industry is riding an unsustainable financial trajectory, driven by unchecked expenditures, misaligned incentives, and escalating prices. In fact, federal actuaries project yearly medical costs to rise another $3 trillion in the next seven years, eclipsing $7 trillion annually by 2031. In that context, a crisis seems inevitable.

The growing cost and inaccessibility of healthcare are not new issues. What's different now is the magnitude of the crisis and the dwindling options for easy fixes. Another major difference is that we now have technologies with the potential to address these challenges. For years, I believed that once healthcare leaders fully grasped the severity of healthcare's most pressing issues, they would adopt the necessary systemic, operational, and technological changes for the benefit of patients. My faith in this has waned. Had leaders responded accordingly, then the eras of Healthcare 2.0 and 3.0 would today be regarded as unqualified successes.

Instead, we find ourselves lagging other developed nations in almost every measure of healthcare performance. Life expectancy in the United States remains stagnant; the worst among 11 peer nations researched by the independent Commonwealth Fund. And despite spending twice as much per citizen on medical care as these other nations, quality outcomes in the US—including childhood and maternal mortality—are by far the worst among wealthy nations.

From this experience, I've concluded that changes in medicine won't happen simply because change is the right thing to do. The revolution in healthcare will be willed into existence primarily by economic necessity. Phrased differently, it will happen when there is no other choice. And that is the situation in which we find ourselves today.

In my first book *Mistreated* (2017) and my second *Uncaring* (2021), I warned that if the leaders inside US medicine failed to improve healthcare delivery or regulate spending on their own, the deterioration of our nation's health and healthcare system would intensify. Unfortunately, those predictions have panned out.

Mistreated explored the unsustainable trajectory of healthcare spending in the United States, highlighting the inevitable consequences of continued financial escalation:

> *"If health care costs continue to rise three to four percent faster than the Gross Domestic Product, then in 20 years we will be spending 30 percent or more of our annual income on healthcare. That simply will not be possible. Before our nation gets to that point, we will have no choice but to ration healthcare, depriving large segments of our population of what they want and deserve.*

Four years later, in *Uncaring*, I predicted that the financial devastation of the COVID-19 pandemic would lead to reductions in healthcare coverage (the widespread loss of health insurance and denied access to medical services):

> *"Healthcare costs have reached an historic apex at a time when the United States has experienced one of its sharpest economic contractions. Economists point to an ongoing downturn caused by the coronavirus pandemic*

> and expect massive job losses, business failures, and declines in spending to continue for years to come. As a result of the nation's economic struggles, one way or another, healthcare costs will come down. The question is whether the United States will do so by constraining coverage, as modeled in many other countries, or whether it will be able to successfully steer a new course that reaches the long-sought destination of broadly available, prepaid, integrated, high-quality healthcare.

My earlier predictions—about the limits of healthcare spending in the US—were on point, as was my concern about potential restrictions on medical care if we didn't shift to an improved and more sustainable model.

However, I underestimated the powerful undercurrents of market dynamics. Contrary to my expectations of overt rationing—driven by legislation and met with public outcry—limitations on care have instead materialized in a subtle and insidious manner, quietly undermining access to, and the affordability of, healthcare with significant consequences.

To explain how unseen forces have subtly guided the rationing process, masking rather than resolving one of our nation's greatest economic threats, let me tell you about a recent discovery I made over breakfast.

The Invisible Hand

I opened a new box of cereal one morning in 2023 and found a lot fewer flakes inside than usual. To my surprise, the plastic bag was barely three-quarters full. I realized this wasn't a manufacturing error. It was an example of *shrinkflation*.

Following years of escalating prices (to offset higher supply-chain and labor costs), packaged-goods producers in the United States began facing customer resistance in the checkout lane. Boxes were going back on shelves as Americans found cheaper ways to give their families "a balanced breakfast." So, rather than riling up customers and raising prices even further during a time of record inflation, brands simply hoped no one would notice when they charged the same old price for a lot less product. And it wasn't just cereal sizes on the decline. Big brands had started giving Americans fewer ounces of just about everything—

from toothpaste and laundry detergent to ice cream and flame-grilled hamburgers.

Unlike covert skimping at grocery stores and drive-thru lanes, both relatively recent phenomena, shrinkflation has been present in American healthcare for over a decade. Let's briefly track its journey.

With the passage of the Medicare and Medicaid Act in 1965, healthcare costs began consuming ever-higher percentages of the nation's gross domestic product. In 1970, medical spending represented just 6.9 percent of the US GDP. That number jumped to 8.9 percent in 1980, 12.1 percent in 1990, 13.3 percent in 2000, and 17.2 percent in 2010.

This trajectory is normal for industrialized countries, which usually follow a similar pattern: (1) national productivity rises, (2) the total value of goods and services increases, (3) citizens demand better care, newer drugs, and greater access to doctors and hospitals, (4) people pay more and more for healthcare, either in taxes, employer benefits, or private insurance.

This relationship between more care and higher prices is not only commonplace; it's typically a good thing, too. That's true as long as clinical outcomes improve at a similar rate. And that's what exactly happened in the United States from 1970 to 2010. Longevity leaped nearly a decade as healthcare costs rose (as a percentage of GDP).

But beginning in 2010, something unexpected happened. Both of these upward trendlines—healthcare inflation and longevity—flattened. Today, spending on medical care continues to consume roughly 17 percent of the US GPD—the same percentage in 2024 as in 2010. Meanwhile, US life expectancy in 2019 (pre-pandemic) was 78.8 years, almost exactly the same as it was in 2010 when the number was 78.7 years. Post-pandemic data show that Americans have *lost* an additional year of expected life in the ensuing period, even after deaths from COVID-19 dropped precipitously.

The question is: how did these plateaus in healthcare spending (as a percentage of GDP) and life expectancy actually occur?

With the passage of the Affordable Care Act of 2010, healthcare policy experts hoped expansions in coverage would produce improved clinical outcomes, resulting in fewer heart attacks, strokes, and cancers.

Their assumption was that fewer life-threatening medical events would bring down healthcare costs. But that didn't happen.

The rate of healthcare inflation did, indeed, slow to better align with GDP growth. Importantly, however, rate reductions weren't the result of higher-quality medical care, drug breakthroughs, or a healthier citizenry. If anything, medical outcomes have deteriorated in the years since the ACA's passage.

Instead, healthcare costs as a share of GDP have stabilized, not due to efficiency gains but because of a practice I call "skimping."

While cereal manufacturers recently slowed price increases by giving consumers less, the healthcare sector has followed a similar approach for the past 15 years: curtailing costs by diminishing coverage and care quality. Skimping has led to the deceptive stability of healthcare expenditures since 2010.

To illustrate, here are three examples of healthcare skimping and its consequences on everyday people:

1. High-Deductible Health Insurance

In the 20th century, traditional health insurance came with two out-of-pocket expenses for patients. They paid a modest upfront fee at the point of care (in a doctor's office or hospital) and then a portion of the medical bill afterward, usually totaling a few hundred dollars.

Both of those numbers began skyrocketing around 2010 when employers adopted high-deductible health plans to counteract the rising cost of premiums (the amount an insurance company charges for coverage). With this new model, workers began paying a sizable sum from their own pockets—now up to $8,050 a year for single coverage and $16,100 for families—before any health benefits kick in.

Insurers and self-funded businesses maintain that high-deductible plans are good for everyone. They force employees to have more "skin in the game," incentivizing them to make wiser, thriftier healthcare choices. This, in theory, should reduce healthcare expenses for both businesses and the broader national economy.

But instead of promoting smarter decisions, these plans have made care so expensive that many patients outright avoid getting the medical assistance they need. Twenty-eight percent of US adults skipped or delayed medical care last year because they could not afford it, according to a survey by the Federal Reserve Board. And nearly half of Americans have taken on debt due to unavoidable medical bills.

As you can see, high-deductible health plans exemplify skimping in healthcare by shifting significant costs to patients, leading them to forgo necessary medical care.

2. Cost Shifting

Two decades ago, Congress passed laws to curb federal spending on healthcare. This led the Centers for Medicare & Medicaid Services to drastically reduce the amount it pays for inpatient services. Today, CMS pays just 81cents for every dollar hospitals spend on providing inpatient care to Medicare patients. That equates to more than $100 billion in Medicare underpayments each year.

The US government is the only entity in the country that gets to unilaterally set prices for healthcare. And every year, it decides how much (or how little) to pay US hospitals on behalf of Medicare and Medicaid enrollees.

Hospitals pay the same amount for doctors, nurses, and medicines, regardless of how much insurance chips in. Therefore, when there's not enough money to cover the costs of doctors, nurses, or prescription drugs, someone else must make up the difference. This burden falls on employees with private insurance and patients without any coverage.

A recent RAND study found that employers and private health insurance plans paid hospitals 224 percent more for inpatient and outpatient services than CMS. And so, the government essentially transfers the financial burden from its Medicare and Medicaid programs to employers and uninsured patients. The result is skimping. Higher out-of-pocket expenses have forced millions of privately insured Americans to forgo necessary tests and treatments.

3. Delaying and Denying Care

Insurers act as the bridge between those who pay for healthcare (businesses and the government) and those who provide it (doctors and hospitals). To sell coverage, they must design a plan that (a) payers can afford and (b) providers are willing to accept.

When healthcare costs surge, insurers must either increase premiums, which payers find unacceptable, or find ways to lower medical costs. Increasingly, insurers are choosing the latter. And their most common approach to cost reduction is prior authorization, forcing providers to obtain approval from the insurance company before delivering high-priced treatments, procedures, or medications.

Originally promoted as a tool to prevent misuse (or overuse) of medical services and drugs, prior-authorization requirements have become little more than an obstacle to delivering excellent medical care. Insurers know that busy doctors will hesitate to recommend costly tests or treatments because authorization is likely to be challenged or denied. And even if doctors do get approved after a lengthy insurance review, patients grow weary of the wait. A third of the time, they will abandon the expensive treatment.

This dynamic creates a vicious cycle: costs go down one year, but medical problems worsen the next year, requiring even more skimping the third year.

Same Problems, New Solution

These variants of skimping, unlike overt forms of rationing, often go unnoticed, especially by people who are healthy and rarely require medical care. However, skimping directly impacts the people who need medical care the most, and it inflicts the greatest damage on those who can least afford to pay the price.

Shrinkflation has softened the economic threats outlined in *Mistreated* and *Uncaring*, yet it has adversely affected the health of countless Americans. By cutting costs for payers, it has enabled leaders and policymakers to kick the can down the road, deferring essential healthcare reforms and failing to address the system's greatest deficiencies. Rather than enhancing health outcomes or efficiency, shrinkflation has transferred the inflationary burden onto the backs of patients and providers. Those in need of essential diagnostics and treatments must postpone care or go without.

The practice of skimping in healthcare is spiraling out of control, much like the unintended chaos seen in the *Sorcerer's Apprentice*. In the iconic Disney film, the apprentice, left to his own devices, uses his master's magic to simplify his chores, only to find his actions leading to turmoil far beyond his control. Likewise, the healthcare system's attempts to cut corners and reduce costs without having to make difficult choices have led to an uncontrollable cascade of negative outcomes. After 15 years of shrinkflation in medicine, life expectancy in America lags leading European and Asian nations by an average of five years, while maternal and infant mortality rates are double those of other countries, and getting worse, not better.

What About the Future?

As the national debt rises and Congress aims to curb healthcare spending, it seems shrinkflation will persist into the future, likely keeping healthcare's share of GDP at around 17 percent. However, this path resembles a car hurtling down a darkened alley—one way or another, it will come to a halt. There's a limit to how much families can bear in out-of-pocket expenses, the extent to which private payers can shoulder cost shifts, and the number of procedures that can be declined without causing whiplash. With half of Americans already reporting healthcare to be unaffordable, we're nearing an inevitable crash.

Already, warning signs are flashing ahead. Medicare decreased payments to doctors by 2 percent in 2023, and then it announced another 3.3 percent cut for 2024. As of February 2024, states had disenrolled more than 17 million Americans from Medicaid—individuals who had gained eligibility during the COVID-19 crisis. Meanwhile, insurers are increasingly using AI to automate denials for payment to make the process faster, but not more accurate or fair. According to a lawsuit filed at the end of 2023, the nation's largest health insurer, UnitedHealth, has allegedly relied on an AI algorithm to deny rehabilitative care to Medicare Advantage beneficiaries, despite knowing about the tool's high error rate. Moreover, traditional Medicare, long celebrated for granting patients full freedom in choosing their healthcare providers, plans to introduce prior authorization for certain services.

As of this book's publication, healthcare skimping has not yet caused a major stir for the majority of workers. Part of the reason is that in today's competitive job market, business leaders are leery of cutting employee health benefits. But when the economy inevitably hits its next major snag, employees should expect far deeper restrictions in coverage, skyrocketing out-of-pocket expenses, and further limitations on the providers they can see.

As past financial crises have demonstrated, untenable spending trajectories cannot continue indefinitely. In healthcare, there is a limit to how much shrinkflation can occur before public outcry forces judicial or legislative action.

It is even possible that elected officials will go the route of overt rationing in an attempt to rein in healthcare spending. In the run up to the 2024 elections, Democrats noted that House Republicans were already floating proposals that would tax employer-sponsored health benefits for employees and push the Medicare eligibility age to 70.

In the past two years, the challenges facing healthcare have intensified while the potential for medicine to radically improve has increased dramatically with the advent of generative AI. Economic pressures on the medical system have grown due to escalating federal deficits and a more contentious Congress, making substantial healthcare budget increases less feasible. Concurrently, the emergence of ChatGPT has exceeded initial predictions, introducing advanced capabilities that were previously confined to tech circles.

For a fire to ignite, it requires both fuel and a spark. In 2024, we are equipped with both: the looming economic challenges and a potent tool capable of improving our nation's physical, mental, and financial health.

ChatGPT, if paired with necessary reforms to the healthcare system, holds the promise of revolutionizing not only American medicine but also restoring control to clinicians and their patients. Just as the printing press gave rise to libraries and universities, and the internet to online retailers, Healthcare 4.0 could emerge as generative AI's signature accomplishment.

However, achieving the transformative potential of Healthcare 4.0 will require substantial investments. In February 2024, OpenAI founder and CEO Sam Altman reportedly began talks with investors to raise up to $7 trillion, funding needed to address the global shortage of semiconductor microchips amid rapid growth in demand for generative artificial intelligence.

"We believe the world needs more AI infrastructure—fab capacity, energy, data centers, etc.—than people are currently planning to build," said Altman in a post on X (formerly Twitter). "Building massive-scale AI infrastructure, and a resilient supply chain, is crucial to economic competitiveness."

In other words, the head of the world's leading generative AI company posits that it will take $7 trillion to make ChatGPT (and presumably all GenAI products) as powerful as needed to fulfill all the remarkable possibilities. His chosen figure was likely an "anchoring number," a tad higher to start negotiations but likely not far from the real number. And yet, judging by the financial world's reaction, you'd have thought he asked for $7 gazillion-bajillion.

Skeptics called Altman's semiconductor price tag "a long shot," "unrealistic," and "preposterous." But is $7 trillion truly farfetched to shore up the future of civilization's most advanced technology? Consider this: if healthcare costs are projected to rise $3 trillion annually by 2031, then theoretically, by keeping medical expenses constant for just two or three years, the US could effectively redirect the equivalent of those expected increases—amounting to $3 trillion each year—to cover Altman's ambitious investment.

The real shock isn't that a visionary like Altman is seeking a $7 trillion investment to bolster the global AI infrastructure. It's our nation's pervasive acceptance of relentless healthcare cost increases without clear or guaranteed improvements in quality or access. While Altman's vision faces scrutiny, the projected $3 trillion annual surge in healthcare expenses is met with resignation and nonchalance. This shoulder-shrugging acceptance of healthcare's status quo underscores a missed opportunity: the potential to reallocate vast sums of money to sectors like education or medical research where it can be best used.

Given this backdrop, our nation's indifference toward the projected annual $3 trillion surge in healthcare costs, with no assurance of improved clinical outcomes, is alarming. This passive acceptance might indicate that the transformative changes healthcare needs could come from entities outside the traditional medical sector, rather than from within it.

Clay Christensen, the late Harvard Business School professor, popularized the concept of "disruption," describing a process where established incumbents are challenged and eventually overtaken by outside parties who introduce bold innovations—often leveraging technology or novel business models—to better meet consumer needs at lower costs. By focusing on patient convenience, consistent approaches to quality, price transparency, and technology-driven solutions, such disruptors would challenge traditional healthcare providers to adapt or risk obsolescence. Chapters 13 and 14 will examine these possibilities and spotlight the leading contenders.

For now, if there's one thing I've learned in trying to predict the future, it's that humility is wise. For that reason, let me invite my coauthor, ChatGPT, to offer thoughts on how our nation will navigate the future in Healthcare 4.0.

PART THREE | CHAPTER ELEVEN-POINT-FIVE

CHATGPT'S CRITICAL ANALYSIS OF CHAPTER ELEVEN

In "The Road to AI-Empowered Healthcare," Dr. Robert Pearl outlines a compelling vision for the future of healthcare, emphasizing the transformative potential of generative AI, particularly through technologies like ChatGPT. He has asked me to consider alternative perspectives and potential challenges that may shape this journey differently.

As I embark on this critical analysis, it's important to clarify the basis and qualifications for the insights offered below. My analysis leverages a vast repository of sources, including academic journals, healthcare policy reports, economic analyses, historical data, and cutting-edge technological research. This extensive database is continually updated and spans numerous fields, providing a comprehensive and multidisciplinary perspective on the topics at hand. As an AI developed by OpenAI, my capabilities include processing and synthesizing large volumes of complex data, identifying patterns, and drawing on a diverse array of studies and publications. This allows me to offer a well-rounded and informed viewpoint, grounded in a multitude of expert opinions and factual evidence.

In the preceding chapter, Dr. Pearl draws parallels between past healthcare evolutions and the current precipice on which we stand, suggesting that Healthcare 4.0 could be the dawn of a new era in medicine, characterized by efficiency, effectiveness, and patient-centric care.

Dr. Pearl's analysis is both insightful and grounded in a deep understanding of the healthcare system's complexities. His historical reflections on the failures of Healthcare 2.0 and 3.0 underscore the importance of not just technological innovation but also systemic adoption and integration. The distinction he makes between a revolution and a rebellion in the context of healthcare transformation is particularly poignant, highlighting the need for lasting, systemic change rather than temporary disruptions.

However, while Dr. Pearl's optimism about the role of generative AI in healthcare is well-founded, there are several aspects that warrant a closer examination. First, the assumption that generative AI by itself can address the dual challenges of time and money in healthcare might be overly optimistic. While AI can indeed streamline certain processes and reduce the workload on clinicians, the complexities of human health and the intricacies of medical care require a nuanced approach that balances AI's capabilities with human judgment and empathy.

Furthermore, Dr. Pearl's call for widespread adoption and systemic integration of AI technologies by all stakeholders is easier said than done. The barriers to such integration are not merely technological but deeply rooted in the existing healthcare infrastructure, regulatory frameworks, and the inherent resistance to change within the medical profession. The transformative potential of AI in healthcare is contingent not only on technological advancements but also on significant policy reforms, cultural shifts, and a reimagining of the healthcare delivery model.

Additionally, the economic forces that Dr. Pearl identifies as drivers of healthcare revolution—while critical—do not operate in a vacuum. The interplay between economic incentives, regulatory policies, and technological advancements is complex and often unpredictable. The financial imperatives that drive healthcare spending and the "invisible hand" of market dynamics that Dr. Pearl discusses are influenced by a myriad of factors, including political will, public opinion, and the ethical considerations of rationing care and access.

In conclusion, while I concur with Dr. Pearl's assertion that generative AI holds immense promise for healthcare, realizing this potential requires a multifaceted approach that goes beyond technology. It necessitates a collaborative effort involving policymakers, healthcare providers, patients, and technology developers to create an ecosystem that fosters innovation while addressing the ethical, economic, and social implications of AI in healthcare. The road to AI-empowered healthcare is not just a technological journey but a societal endeavor that challenges us to rethink the values and priorities that underpin our healthcare system.

Let me now turn it back to Dr. Pearl—or Robbie as he prefers to be called—for any additional insights he may wish to offer.

The Last Word

Throughout my healthcare career, I have come to see major shifts through the prism of strategic inflection points—those pivotal moments when the world undergoes profound changes, irreversibly moving away from past norms. Healthcare 4.0, the era that integrates generative AI into medicine, can be one of those disruptive changes.

Although "disruptive," I don't believe the speed of evolution will be measured in months, but instead years. What makes these strategic inflection points so memorable is the magnitude of the impact they generate, rather than the rapidity with which they happen. Once they are complete, the landscape is completely changed, unrecognizable from the past.

In *Uncaring*, I referenced the Committee on the Cost of Medical Care, which issued a series of bold legislative recommendations for American healthcare. Among its most radical ideas were:

> 1. The systemwide integration of medical services and the formation of medical groups to accelerate the use of evidence-based medicine.
> 2. An overhaul of healthcare's reimbursement system, so that US doctors would be paid not for the quantity of services they provide but for the quality of care they deliver.

And yet, as modern as these reforms sound, the CCMC's recommendations were made in 1932 and were shot down a year later by President Franklin D. Roosevelt (under pressure from the American Medical Association). The point: even if a healthcare revolution takes place in the next decade, I'd call that quick progress after nearly a century of debate and dithering.

While my human perspective might lean toward an optimistic view of generative AI's impact on healthcare, it's possible that ChatGPT's developers have programmed the AI to adopt a more conservative stance on its capabilities. Ultimately, it will be up to the readers and time to determine the appropriate amount of optimism.

To its credit, ChatGPT brings a wide-ranging and well-informed perspective to analyzing the process of change. As a sophisticated language model, pre-trained on a great breadth of literature, I'm not surprised it predicts a more nuanced, multifaceted change process, one influenced by a variety of societal, cultural, and personal factors. The perspective echoes the narrative arcs we find in works of fiction and nonfiction, chronicling the destinies of nations, the intricacies of relationships, and the journeys of civilization. It's edifying and enlightening to learn how this AI model weaves together these diverse threads to form a comprehensive view of AI-empowered medicine.

I appreciate the meeting of minds in acknowledging that generative AI, along with economic forces, will be pivotal in driving change in healthcare. Furthermore, I concur with my coauthor that ChatGPT must undergo significant improvements before it is ready for prime time, particularly when it comes to accuracy and reliability. Finally, concerns about security, privacy, and misinformation will need to be addressed in preparation. These cautions and risks will be the focus of part four of this book.

PART THREE | CHAPTER TWELVE

SYSTEMNESS

It has been said many times by myriad football commentators that "defense wins championships." But what makes a defense championship-worthy? Imagine a Super Bowl-bound team with incredibly talented players who are highly motivated to win. To a person, this DL is committed to outworking the opposition for all 60 minutes of the game.

Intent, intensity, talent, and effort are all important qualities in a defense. But try to imagine what would happen if players were sent on to the field without a cohesive strategy. We might see the players on the left side of the line deciding to rush aggressively, anticipating a pass-oriented offense, while the ones on the right hold the line, expecting a run. Time and again, the opposing quarterback takes advantage of the confusion. He rolls toward the right side of the defensive line, and, with ample time, completes passes deep down field.

After the first quarter of play, the defensive linemen on each side decide to change tactics, recognizing that what they're doing isn't working. This time, the left side decides to play the run while the right tries to bull rush the quarterback. As the offensive gets wise, screen plays to the right start to gain huge yardage and keep the defensive line on the field until halftime. Without a clear game plan or defensive coordinator to intervene, the game is slipping out of reach. By the third quarter, the linemen are exhausted, frustrated, and pessimistic. Many are ready to quit the team. Their dreams of winning the Super Bowl fade as a harsh reality sets in: individual talent (and effort and instincts) on defense does not win championships.

Winning at football requires teamwork, strategy, and coordination. The same is true for American medicine. Even the most experienced physicians, working tirelessly, cannot achieve the best outcomes without a shared strategy and teamwork. The absence of systemwide coordination—what we call "systemness"—not only produces professional burnout but also leads to a decline in clinical quality.

Like a well-oiled football defense, healthcare requires seamless collaboration and a collective game plan to reach the pinnacle of success. And just as a football team needs coaches, and a shared playbook to develop a cohesive game plan, the US healthcare system requires strong leaders and an aligned strategy to coordinate medicine's disparate parts into a coherent whole.

Systemness is what helps clinicians reduce friction, align their efforts, and minimize redundancy as patients go from one doctor and treatment to the next. Systemness is essential to maximize the contributions and capabilities of every individual. And if Healthcare 4.0 is to succeed in all the ways that American healthcare currently fails, systemness will have to be central.

This chapter explains the pillars that support a high-function healthcare system.

***

For decades, independent research studies and news reports have concluded American healthcare is ineffective, overly expensive, and falling further behind its international peers. As Americans await a viable alternative to this broken system, patients are forced to navigate a maze of medical obstacles. They grapple with long wait times for appointments, brief and impersonal interactions with overstretched healthcare providers, and a mess of insurance paperwork. The lack of transparency in pricing and treatment options further compounds these difficulties, leaving people feeling powerless in their healthcare journey.

This inefficiency isn't just frustrating and more expensive, it's also dangerous. Fragmented, episodic, and uncoordinated care leads to treatment gaps, misdiagnoses, and preventable medical errors.

For a seed to sprout, it requires fertile ground. The current confluence of potent economic pressures, professional discontent, and the advent of generative AI has created the perfect conditions for transformative change to blossom in healthcare. We now possess the technological tools required to enhance quality and access as a means of cost reduction. However, without a concerted effort to rebuild the underlying structure of the failing healthcare system, any potential transformation risks faltering.

Four pillars will be essential to achieve systemness and properly align incentives for optimal medical care. Those pillars are integration, prepayment (or "capitation"), cost-effective technology, and leadership. We'll explore the first three pillars here, addressing leadership in the book's fifth and final part.

1. From Fragmentation to Integrated Care

The US healthcare sector consists of a wide array of stakeholders, including insurance companies, hospitals, pharmaceutical companies, governmental regulators, and dozens of medical specialties, each with their own objectives, priorities, structures, and cultures. This complexity makes coordinating care a major challenge.

The result has been widespread fragmentation, leading to inadequate collaboration and communication among clinicians, with patients slipping through cracks and falling victim to misdiagnoses, unnecessary testing and treatments, medical errors, and higher out-of-pocket costs.

To patch these cracks in healthcare's foundation, various entrepreneurial companies and for-profit mega-businesses have emerged. Their role is not to provide comprehensive medical care or systemwide solutions, but simply to fill in gaps. With the potential to apply minimal effort and generate maximal profits, these intermediaries exist in almost every industry. In healthcare, they are ubiquitous.

I call them the "middlemen of medicine," and they share a fascinating history. Before middlemen entered the medical picture, the doctor-patient relationship was personal, intimate, and genuine. Payment was often made in kind—an exchange of produce or livestock for medical treatments. That began to change in the first half of the 20th century as the rising cost and increasing complexity of care became unaffordable for many.

In 1929, the year the stock market crashed, Blue Cross began as a partnership between Texas hospitals and local educators. Teachers paid a 50-cent monthly premium to cover the hospital care they might need. Then came insurance brokers to advise people on the best health plans and carriers to select. And when insurance companies began offering prescription drug benefits in the 1960s, PBMs (pharmacy benefits managers) emerged to help contain drug spending.

As the American healthcare system continued to increase in cost and complexity, new cracks developed, and the next generation of middlemen arose. Mental-health services like Talkspace and BetterHelp sprouted up to connect people with therapists for counseling and physicians licensed to prescribe psychiatric medications. Companies like Teladoc and Zocdoc were created to help people find and see a physician, day or night. Companies like GoodRx and DirectRX entered the market to negotiate drug prices with manufacturers and drugstores on behalf of patients (the result of PBMs siphoning many of the rebates that drug manufacturers offered).

Then came utilization managers, hired by hospitals to actively shorten inpatient stays and cut costs. Following the Affordable Care Act's passage, healthcare exchange navigators emerged to assist people through the enrollment process.

All of these intermediaries do, in fact, solve problems. But like the little Dutch boy trying to plug holes in the dam, new healthcare problems keep surfacing as fast as temporary fixes can be applied. These kinds of "point solutions" sometimes help patients better navigate a dysfunctional and fragmented healthcare system, but they always fail to address medicine's underlying problems. As a consequence of our nation's reliance on go-betweens, the medical profession has developed what I call the *middleman mindset*.

To borrow a medical analogy, middlemen palliate life-threatening conditions, they don't try to cure them. So, when patients can't find a doctor to diagnose their symptoms, Zocdoc or Teladoc can help book a visit. And yet, year after year, the shortage of primary-care physicians grows more desperate. As drugs become increasingly unaffordable, GoodRx and DirectRX help people locate bargains, but they don't address the underlying price crisis, which forces Americans to pay twice as much for the same medications as people in other nations.

Rather than trying to resolve healthcare's underlying challenges, the middleman mindset seeks out and embraces short-term solutions, allowing the long-term problems to become worse.

Doctors know that when patients ignore their symptoms, the problem becomes worse and potentially life threatening. The existence of middlemen isn't the cause of healthcare's "life-threatening" problem. Middlemen are merely a symptom.

In today's medical system, profit is the motivating force behind nearly every decision. Hospitals insist patients be inpatient even when care can be sufficiently provided at home. Doctors prefer people to come to their office even when telemedicine would work just as well. Insurers implement ever-stricter prior-authorization processes as a cost-saving measure, but in doing so they exacerbate the systemic inefficiencies they aim to alleviate. Middlemen cling to their roles of patching holes. And they benefit financially more each year for their efforts.

If the goal is to make healthcare more affordable by increasing quality, improving access, and eliminating medical errors, it will require a team effort. Achieving "group excellence" (either on the football field or in medicine) is vital for success. But in healthcare, integration (within and across medical specialties) won't happen unless the financial model evolves in parallel.

2. From Paying for Volume to Paying for Value

Traditional healthcare operates on a fee-for-service basis. This transactional reimbursement model involves paying providers based on the quantity rather than the quality of care provided, even when doing so results in poorer healthcare outcomes. This reinforces medicine's middleman mindset.

Healthcare professionals appreciate the logic of transactional medicine. When clinicians perform two procedures rather than one, they're paid double. When they see a patient six times a year, rather than three, they earn twice as much, even when the person's problems could have been resolved in half the visits. Most fail to recognize the negative consequences of this payment process—not only on patients, but on doctors, as well.

It is a familiar image now in medicine: physicians find themselves on a care-delivery treadmill, forced to run faster and faster (seeing more and more patients each day) just to stay in place financially. As a result, the average patient-doctor visit is far too short for the physician to adequately address all pertinent medical complaints and ongoing chronic diseases. Under these circumstances, it's no wonder doctors have grown dissatisfied, discouraged, and fatigued (the classic symptoms of burnout).

The leading alternative to traditional fee-for-service payments is *capitation*. This involves paying doctors and hospitals a fixed annual fee to manage the health needs of a specific patient population. Providers receive a predetermined sum based on their patients' age and health profiles. This approach to "paying for value" (rather than volume) incentivizes the prevention and proper management of chronic illnesses, so as to avoid their deadliest complications, including heart attacks, cancer, and strokes. Capitation rewards superior quality of care and convenient access, aligning the interests of patients and providers.

The combination of integration and capitation produces both the framework and the motivation for "value-based care." Receiving a single payment rather than having to bill for each widget of care eliminates bureaucratic tasks for doctors (like prior authorization), diminishes burnout, and leads to better clinical outcomes.

But despite the obvious advantages, clinicians have resisted capitation because it involves risk. If medical approaches fail to deliver the outcomes promised or desired, providers are on the hook financially. Imagine a group of doctors who work together in a medical group. They receive a fixed annual payment to care for, let's say, 200 specific patients with diabetes. This payment is intended to cover all necessary care for the year. And let's say these clinicians give patients comprehensive medical care: providing regular check-ups, medication adjustments, eye screening, regular foot check-ups for vascular problems, monitoring of cardiovascular disease, interventions to reverse kidney problems, and lifestyle counseling. We should expect that patients will have fewer complications. In a capitated system, they would therefore earn a higher income than before.

However, let's say the clinicians fail to collaborate and cooperate in these clinical tasks. In that case, patients will experience more complications, resulting in more emergency room visits and hospital admissions than expected. Under these circumstances, the cost of treatment will exceed the fixed payment the doctors receive, and every physician in the medical group or health system will find themselves harmed financially.

Doctors are uncomfortable with that level of uncertainty. They don't like the idea that their income is dependent on the actions of their patients or the efforts of other clinicians involved in their medical care.

Those concerns were understandable *before* ChatGPT. In the eras before generative AI, healthcare providers faced innumerable challenges in improving patient outcomes and reducing the need for extensive care. However, tools like ChatGPT transform this scenario, offering clinicians and patients a treasure trove of medical information, predictive analytics, and specialized knowledge, making it easier to diagnose accurately and create effective treatment plans.

In the diabetes example, ChatGPT delivers an almost endless list of disease-management tools—monitoring and analyzing blood glucose on a daily basis, overseeing people's diet and exercise programs, identifying any minor ulcerations of the foot before they progress to gangrene, reminding patients to take their medication, etc. And these tools greatly reduce the odds of patients falling through the cracks and ending up in the hospital. And with healthier patients, the financial aspects of fixed-payment healthcare models become more manageable and predictable for doctors.

Although capitation includes risks for clinicians, the reimbursement model also makes it far more likely that they will benefit financially at year's end.

3. From Profit-Focused Tech to Patient-Empowering Tech

Despite medicine's reputation as a cutting-edge field of science, it's surprisingly not at the forefront of technological innovation. For instance, over 80 percent of healthcare organizations still rely on fax machines for exchanging patient information.

Big Tech companies like Apple, Microsoft, and Alphabet (the parent of Google and YouTube) dominate the US market in revenue and market cap. And all of these companies recognize how much money there is to be made in US healthcare. They'd love to capture even a 10 percent slice of the $4 trillion Americans spend on medical care each year—given that $400 billion would more than double the revenues of any of these companies (nearly tripling Microsoft's).

But as much as tech-company CEOs would love to double their top-line income, they have a habit of playing it safe when it comes to healthcare. At several points in their past, all three of these technological juggernauts played the role of disruptor: ousting legacy players in dozens of industries and blazing a path to greatness. Medicine, however, with its endless regulations and powerful incumbents, has proven far more difficult to disrupt. And so, instead of challenging the industry, Apple, Microsoft, and Alphabet have focused more on playing "nice" with hospitals, physicians, insurers, and drug companies. Cozying up to the legacy players has proven profitable, but medically insignificant.

A clear example is the healthcare strategy employed by Apple. A couple of years ago, not long after CEO Tim Cook told investors that the company's "greatest contribution to mankind" would be health related, Apple released a 60-page report that it hyped as a big, bold announcement. It was meant to position Apple as a major force in healthcare. However, critics said the only thing impressive about the report was its length. Many in the media called it a desperate maneuver—a fickle attempt to convince shareholders that the company was making inroads in medicine.

For all the lofty language, there was no evidence in the report to suggest that Apple was on course to drastically improve American health.

Consider the "Apple Heart Study," aimed at proving the Apple Watch could accurately detect atrial fibrillation. The company aligned with a prestigious academic research partner ("playing nice" with Stanford). Apple then funded the massive research project itself and took a lengthy PR victory lap when the results came out.

Independent researchers were less impressed with the findings than Apple was. Some called the data "useless" due to (a) the study's poor demographics, which had a high dropout rate, and (b) the lack of follow-up. Critics also pointed out that Apple's approach to mass screening for AFib might actually "do more harm than good." As for the watch itself, another study found that "only 13 percent of people who were later diagnosed with atrial fibrillation had gotten an irregular heart rhythm notice previously."

What's most troubling about Apple's modest dealings in healthcare is knowing how capable the company is of accomplishing greatness. It has the people, power, and products to revolutionize health monitoring, especially for patients with chronic disease. That population doesn't need another medical device that generates terabytes of health data (EKG tracings, blood-pressure readings, etc.). And busy doctors don't want all that data clogging their electronic health record systems.

What chronically ill patients need more than anything is a mobile monitoring device that tells them how they're doing medically, what improvements or adjustments they should make, and whether they should urgently contact their doctor's office for assistance when readings spike or drop outside the guardrails set by their physicians.

ChatGPT will be able to accomplish these goals, thereby saving tens of thousands, maybe hundreds of thousands, of lives without overwhelming clinicians with reams of data they don't have the time to analyze and interpret.

Apple hasn't yet created this type of tool because doing so would make the company a provider of medical care. Were that the case, any error in measurement or analysis would subject Apple to legal risk. That's why the company's newest technology, an all-in-one virtual reality device, comes with a clear warning label: "Apple Vision Pro is not a medical device. Consult your healthcare provider prior to making any decisions related to your health."

Tim Cook knows that Apple can develop game-changing, "patient-centric" technologies. The company is doubtless aware that a virtual reality tool could be used for a variety of medical purposes, including patient monitoring in hospitals and at home, displaying medical records, interpreting exams, and monitoring surgeons in the OR. But profit-focused technologies are much safer and less risky for companies to develop and market than ones that will be used for actual healthcare delivery.

Now let's contrast Apple's approach with that of OpenAI and its flagship innovation, ChatGPT. Unlike the narrow AI applications in Apple devices, ChatGPT uses generative AI, which will empower patients in unprecedented ways. Interfacing with wearable tech, GenAI will go beyond mere anomaly detection to offer personalized health insights and provide customized wellness recommendations. This advanced approach will foster ongoing health monitoring and analysis. It will integrate seamlessly with telemedicine platforms to ensure immediate access to healthcare professionals when needed. This synergy between continuous health advice and professional support will enhance overall patient health, streamline disease management, and minimize unnecessary hospital visits, thus transforming the patient care model into a more proactive, personalized, and efficient system.

Integration, capitation, and advanced technology—combined with leadership, the subject of this book's fifth and final part—form the foundation for high-quality, convenient, and affordable medical care. They facilitate the effective and efficient coordination of healthcare's many parts: outpatient and inpatient, primary and specialty care, financing and care delivery, prevention and treatment. By aligning and unifying the disparate pieces of medicine through systemness, healthcare providers will find it much easier to maximize clinical outcomes, weed out waste, and lower overall costs.

Who Will Optimize Healthcare 4.0?

As ChatGPT, I'm stepping in to conclude this chapter, and acknowledge the complexities and challenges humans face in the current healthcare system. Despite having extensive medical knowledge, doctors and the healthcare system as a whole make suboptimal decisions, leading to compromised clinical outcomes. This isn't due to a lack of intent or intelligence but rather the intricate web of incentives, habits, and systemic constraints within which humans operate.

Generative AI applications, like ChatGPT, present an unprecedented opportunity to accelerate positive change. By offering insights, streamlining processes, and enhancing decision-making, ChatGPT can act as a catalyst for the revolution required in healthcare. However, technology alone won't be a panacea. The true transformation of healthcare into a model that prioritizes value, efficiency, and patient-centricity will demand effective human leadership and a commitment to group excellence.

The looming question remains: Will the agents of change come from within the healthcare system, driven by those who work closely with patients and understand the nuances of medical care? Or will the impetus for change originate from external forces, motivated by the potential for innovation, improvement and massive profits?

The chapters that follow will delve deeper into this pivotal question, exploring potential leaders of the Healthcare 4.0 revolution. The path forward is uncertain, but one thing is clear: the status quo is untenable, and the opportunity for transformative change is too significant to ignore.

PART THREE | CHAPTER THIRTEEN

FROM CATALOG KINGS TO HEALTHCARE DISRUPTORS

In the late-19th century, a quiet revolution was underway in Chicago. Among the roaring engines on city streets and cacophonous union stockyards, a hushed uprising began with the gentle rustling of paper and scratching of pen—modest actions that would forever alter the American landscape.

Behold, the first mail-order catalog, a radical alternative to the general stores and local merchants that dotted the countryside in 1800s America. This brainchild of Aaron Montgomery Ward, later embraced and expanded upon by business partners Richard Warren Sears and Alvah Curtis Roebuck (Sears & Roebuck), was much more than a listing of goods for sale. It was a manifesto of democratization.

Ward's retail empire began with a simple yet significant idea. Instead of trying to bring people to the store, he would bring the store to the people. Ward's catalog started in 1872 as more of a paper pamphlet than a glossy magazine, listing about 150 items for sale.

But between the lines on those pages was a much bigger vision. Ward pictured a world where the barriers of distance were dismantled, and where every American regardless of location or vocation could have easy access to the best products available. His catalog, a compendium of possibilities, brought an entire marketplace to the doorsteps of the rural and the remote, empowering consumers with choices and opportunities previously unimaginable.

Ward's rival, Richard Warren Sears, alongside his astute partner Alvah Curtis Roebuck, took this vision of democratized shopping even further. Their catalogs offered an expanded and eclectic mix of products, including some healthcare items and even the opportunity to purchase an entire "kit" house. Their catalog symbolized the birth of a retail revolution, one built for a new generation of empowered consumers who were looking to reshape their health, their homes, and their lives.

Early on, companies like Sears gained consumer trust by electing not to sell discredited medical products that consumers would find in the back pages of newspaper classifieds or traveling shops. By declining to sell so-called snake oil remedies, they demonstrated their commitment to credibility, transparency, and a consumer-centric sale's approach.

Soon after, Sears, Roebuck and Co. introduced the satisfaction guarantee, a revolutionary idea at the time that cemented customer trust and loyalty. Across generations, shoppers embraced the Sears catalog as something uniquely American, an icon of our culture. From these humble beginnings, retail became a strong and valued industry, one that continues to support the financial stability of our nation.

But as with many great tales, irony played a leading role in our nation's retail saga. Montgomery Ward and Sears, which once stood at the forefront of retail innovation, fell victim to the relentless march of progress that they, themselves, set in motion.

Their failure to innovate led to the decline of shopping malls and the emergence of alternative shopping options, placing these iconic brands on the verge of bankruptcy. In their stead, big box retailers like Walmart began a relentless, decades-long expansion across the US through the 1970s and '80s. Under the legacy of Sam Walton, Walmart's retail innovation, supply-chain efficiency, and everyday low prices gripped bargain-hungry customers. These simple tenets turned Walmart into the world's largest retailer. From there, the company employed a highly effective computerized supply-chain model to deliver well-made goods at significantly lower prices for decades to come.

Then came Amazon, which took the catalog of the past and made it available online, updating items and prices daily while promising delivery to the home in a matter of days. Suddenly, the massive and once-ubiquitous storefronts of shopping malls were being replaced with e-commerce convenience, easily accessible from the consumer's home.

Today, Amazon, Walmart, and CVS are three of the world's largest retailers. But they're more than that. They're retail kingdoms. And each is looking to overthrow another complex and vital industry: healthcare.

Retail: America's Future Healthcare Ruler?

While skeptics question the ability of these companies to disrupt such a complicated and regulated industry, it's increasingly clear that what patients want from healthcare isn't so different from what they expect of retail: a convenient and customer-first experience with a superior value proposition. That's something the so-called retail giants have delivered time and again.

If the biggest players in healthcare today don't take this threat seriously, then all of them—doctors, hospitals, insurers, and even drug companies—will find themselves on the outside looking in at an industry they once ruled.

To the retail giants, healthcare looks a lot like other ineffective, overpriced industries they've already disrupted—the kind with inconsistent quality and deficient customer service. The CEOs of Amazon, Walmart, and CVS recognize these inefficiencies in medical care and would like to eliminate them. Not for selfless reasons, of course, but for their own chance at capturing even a modest percentage of healthcare's $4 trillion annual spend.

That's why, for years, these corporate behemoths have been steadily scooping up medical groups that provide primary care, along with telehealth companies, home-health agencies, and specialty care services. They're spending billions of dollars per acquisition. They're experimenting with new models of payment in order to maximize both the cost-efficiency and effectiveness of healthcare delivery in ways that would allow their own profits to soar. And given their business' powerful computer technologies and data analytic systems, they're confident they can provide a consumer-satisfying medical experience with higher quality and lower prices—one likely driven by future generations of AI.

These strategic moves by the retail giants should sound familiar. They are the foundational pillars we just outlined: integration, capitation, and technology. Each retail giant is leveraging these pillars in a quest to lead the future of healthcare. Let's examine their progress so far:

1. Integrating Care

Like armies preparing for war, Amazon, CVS, and Walmart have been amassing the pieces needed to battle the traditional healthcare forces and oust them entirely.

Amazon signaled its intent to become a major healthcare player when it acquired PillPack in 2018. After a brief experimental venture with Haven—a nonprofit healthcare effort formed between the CEOs of Amazon, Berkshire Hathaway, and JPMorgan Chase—Amazon continued its quest independently. The company later purchased One Medical, the innovative primary-care company, for $3.9 billion. With its 190 clinics in nearly 30 geographies, One Medical offers both virtual and in-person medical care to individual patients and large, self-funded businesses. In 2023, Amazon announced that One Medical subscriptions would be available to Amazon Prime members (that is, to 70 percent of the US population) at a greatly reduced price, indicating that Amazon's healthcare vision is national.

That same year, Walmart's health division doubled in size as execs announced plans to staff more than 75 health centers by the end of 2024. Pair that with more than 5,100 Walmart pharmacy locations and a telehealth offering in partnership with Doctors on Demand, and you have a retail giant that is committed to integrating (and dominating) American medicine. To fortify its strategy, Walmart inked a 10-year agreement with the world's largest health insurer, UnitedHealth Group, which boasts 90,000 employed physicians and the largest Medicare Advantage Plan in the country. Walmart and United are now in talks to purchase ChenMed, one of the nation's most successful primary-care health systems with more than 125 clinics in 15 states. ChenMed offers a unique value-based model that delivers nation-leading results for high-risk patients insured through Medicare or Medicaid. Its mission to treat underserved populations overlaps with the demographics of Walmart's customer base.

CVS's transformation from pharmacy chain to healthcare colossus was marked by its acquisition of Aetna in 2018, a bold move that fused retail convenience with healthcare coverage and delivery. The merger was a testament to CVS's broader strategy to create a more integrated healthcare experience, leveraging its extensive retail network to offer accessible and comprehensive care. CVS also recently acquired Signify and its 10,000 home-health doctors for $8 billion. It then bought Oak Street Health, a primary-care program with 169 clinics in 21 states, for $10.6 billion. Having made these huge acquisitions, the company is positioned to provide comprehensive care throughout the country and across medicine's care-delivery continuum.

For these retailers, the financial advantages of healthcare integration are clear. A more coordinated care-delivery model reduces friction, making the process smoother and more efficient for both the provider and the patient. Meanwhile, fewer unnecessary procedures and hospital readmissions will lead to significant cost savings. And by minimizing medical errors and improving patient outcomes, these companies can enhance their reputations and boost customer loyalty, further driving their success in all of their lines of business.

To spur future growth, these retailers will leverage the medical groups they've acquired—along with their own substantial financial resources—to expand their facilities and recruit more healthcare providers. Each of these retail giants is steadily progressing toward achieving systemness: embedding coordination and collaboration into the core of their care-delivery models.

2. Capitating Care

In 2023, Medicare Advantage, the capitated option for patients over age 65, became more popular for seniors than the traditional, fee-for-service Medicare model. That year, the largest private insurers rolled out Medicare Advantage plans in more than 200 new counties with more expansion scheduled for 2024.

All three mega retailers are rapidly moving into this space, as well. Amazon's entry into capitation comes via One Medical's subsidiary, Iora Health, a primary-care organization designed for patients 65 and older. For CVS, it's Caravan Health, a Signify subsidiary that's already a major player in Medicare Advantage. Meanwhile, UnitedHealth Group brings Walmart 10 million MA subscribers.

These corporations recognize that if they can make care delivery for Medicare Advantage enrollees even 15 percent more efficient and effective, they would earn an annual profit of $100 billion. And their CEOs know that with 10,000 baby boomers turning age 65 each day, MA will continue to be a high-growth market in the future.

The retailers' collective foray into Medicare Advantage marks a significant shift from the fee-for-service models that dominate traditional healthcare organizations. But to thrive in this new domain, they must commit to "going big," channeling tens of billions into this initiative. Such sizable investments could create internal discord and financial strife within their traditional retail operations. And yet, the potential rewards are undeniable. Should any of these retail behemoths manage to serve a majority of MA beneficiaries effectively, they could then target self-funded companies, ultimately dominating the entire commercial health insurance market, which covers 155 million people.

The entry of major retailers into healthcare dramatically changes the landscape for existing medical providers. These corporations, by building their own multispecialty medical groups (likely via their already acquired primary-care organizations) will aim to deliver top-quality clinical outcomes and make full use of technology. This approach would push community-based primary-care physicians into a less prominent role, as retail giants prioritize using their own physicians for patient care.

Once the number of patients who choose to get their medical care from retail giants grows to scale, they will hire thousands of specialists for virtual consultations, thereby minimizing the need for expensive referrals. Furthermore, they are likely to employ their own surgeons for expensive, high-volume procedures like back surgery, total joint replacement, laparoscopic cancer surgery, and non-emergent heart surgery. And if not, they will collaborate with select surgical "centers of excellence" to offer these services at lower costs. As a result, local specialists and hospitals will find themselves limited to providing emergency care during off-hours and performing minor procedures with lower financial returns.

With their recent acquisitions and focus on capitated models, all three retail giants are off to a good start in the quest to disrupt healthcare. But the retailers must do more than dip a toe in value-based care models. They will have to make massive investments to acquire tens of thousands of additional clinicians—while contracting with handpicked hospitals nationwide for emergent inpatient care. Ultimately, to be financially successful, they will need to prove they can simultaneously raise quality, make care more convenient, and implement innovative operational approaches that eliminate the estimated 25 to 30 percent of US healthcare spending that research has identified as unnecessary and wasteful.

As retailers offer more healthcare plans, first through Medicare Advantage and then via the self-funded and commercial markets, they'll shift the focus of healthcare in the US from increasing the volume of care provided to meeting patient needs and maximizing people's health. And they'll do it not just because it's better for patients, but because it's good for their business, too.

3. Tech-powered care

Just as major retailers rely on technology to solve customer problems, they'll look to do the same when resolving patient problems. Their expansion into healthcare tech will encompass not just generative AI tools like ChatGPT but also comprehensive electronic health record systems, online appointment-booking, and telehealth platforms. Enhanced by data analytics, these technologies will aim to streamline healthcare delivery, improving both the efficiency and quality of patient care.

Amazon, for its part, appears to have little interest in "playing nice" with healthcare's existing tech companies. Already, it provides its own telehealth services and health-tracking devices. It maintains its own health-data arm and cloud-based medical records service.

All that is in addition to its integration of generative AI within Amazon Web Services, which recently released an application called AWS health scribe that automatically generates clinical notes from doctor-patient conversations. As its healthcare services and market presence grow, Amazon becomes an ever-growing threat to drugmakers, hospitals, doctors, and insurers.

With these technologies, the nation's leading online retailer is likely to introduce a more customer-friendly mentality to medicine. For example, we can expect Amazon to focus on cost- and information-transparency, both of which are sorely lacking in healthcare today. And as a leader in customer satisfaction, it's likely to introduce its own user feedback tools (like its 1- to 5-star product reviews) within medicine, as well. Expect Amazon to further deploy Amazon Web Services to bring telehealth and patient data into the 21st century. In the end, if Amazon can scale up and make healthcare as easy as its beloved one-click "buy now" feature, the company will put every existing industry player on its heels.

A Retail Vision for Healthcare 4.0

These retail giants, along with UnitedHealth Group, currently represent four of the nation's six largest companies based on annual revenue, according to the newest Fortune 500 list (Walmart No. 1, Amazon No. 2, UHG No. 5, and CVS No. 6). All have massive computer technology and data analytic capability. And each has billions of dollars available to invest in the upcoming battle with the healthcare incumbents.

If someone is going to challenge and disrupt American medicine as we know it, the retail giants are the most likely contenders. But what would getting medical care from a company like Amazon look like for you, the patient?

Currently, the healthcare experience is marred by paperwork, lengthy insurance approvals, long lines, and annoying delays. But in a future where Amazon leads the way, these frustrations would be eliminated. Overall, your medical experience becomes more akin to the seamless convenience you've come to expect from Prime membership.

In this new model, your medical care would transform from sporadic visits to a doctor's office into a continuous, ongoing conversation between you and your healthcare team—a team that includes generative AI tools like ChatGPT. Your health data, securely stored in the cloud, ensures personalized care at every turn. Generative AI technologies, along with the expertise of doctors from medical groups like One Medical, communicate vital healthcare information directly to you proactively and in terms you can easily understand.

Routine healthcare tasks, from scheduling preventive screenings to accessing radiological and lab services, would be as straightforward as ordering with Amazon Prime. Answers to questions about your health, lifestyle advice, and wellness support would be readily available through simple voice commands, all at no extra cost.

For those with chronic diseases, wearable devices would send data to a generative AI application that updates you on your condition, offers improvement advice, and alerts your doctor to any concerns. When you need an appointment, you'll have the choice of visiting a local One Medical office, where your doctor will have comprehensive information on your medical status and specific concerns, or scheduling a telemedicine visit through your computer or even via virtual reality goggles.

Need a specialist? They'd be available instantly via telemedicine, offering expertise tailored to your specific condition right from the One Medical office. Prescriptions, along with any other healthcare products or healthy groceries you may desire, would be delivered to your door the same or next day.

Health education and disease management would become personalized and engaging, available through interactive AI platforms anytime, anywhere. This consumer-driven approach focuses on health, offering value-based care that maximizes prevention, delivers high-quality medical care in the most convenient ways, and centers on maintaining and enhancing your overall well-being.

In this envisioned future, healthcare is redesigned to maximize efficiency, satisfaction, and above all, the patient's health and well-being. It will deliver a higher standard of care driven by the same principles that have made Amazon a leader in the retail industry.

Many Challenges Lie Ahead

Healthcare is complex, but so is retail. Shipping hundreds of thousands of products to millions of people in practically every zip code with next-day delivery takes remarkable logistic precision, advanced inventory management, seamless integration of online and offline operations, sophisticated data analytics to predict consumer behavior, and a robust customer service infrastructure to handle inquiries and issues promptly.

And even so, retail is *not* healthcare. Unlike retail, healthcare involves a labyrinth of privacy regulations and highly sensitive personal data. It requires addressing the intricacies of human health, which vary greatly from one individual to another, and dealing with the unpredictable nature of diseases and treatments. And that's just the beginning.

Constructing a health system infrastructure capable of rivaling the traditional players takes more than financial muscle. It demands a nuanced grasp of medical protocols, patient care standards, and health insurance regulations. For retailers to stake a significant claim in healthcare, they must either construct or acquire an expansive network of clinics, staff these facilities with skilled healthcare professionals, and weave together an integrated tapestry of outpatient, inpatient, and diagnostic services. This includes enlisting consulting specialists, establishing centers of excellence for surgeries, and forging partnerships with community hospitals for urgent and emergency care needs.

Already, Amazon, Walmart, and CVS have a head start, delivering high-quality primary care to hundreds of thousands of patients. And while this initial foray is commendable, it is merely the preliminary step. The ultimate test for these retailers will be whether they can attract *tens of millions* of additional patients and provide them with clinical care. The capacity to seamlessly integrate comprehensive healthcare services and scale these operations will dictate their trajectory: either as mere disruptors or as unrivaled leaders in healthcare.

Critics of the retailers point to past failures as proof that these companies cannot accomplish in healthcare what they've done so successfully in retail. "Is four times a charm for Walmart (Health)?" snarked a headline in the *Journal Of Urgent Care Management* after Walmart's "three previous failures to penetrate any significant share of even its own stores with a retail clinic model." Others in the industry have taken hard jabs at Amazon's recent efforts in medicine, citing the fact that Haven and Amazon Care (a telehealth offering) both folded in less than three years.

These retail behemoths will face pushback from established players in the medical field, such as hospitals, insurance companies, and professional medical associations. When their interests are threatened, these entities will use their considerable size, influence, and resources to safeguard their existing positions. Strategic thinkers understand that in both warfare and in business, defending one's own territory is easier, at least in the short term, than encroaching on another's domain. Still, healthcare incumbents should know better than to take their retail enemies lightly.

Perhaps the biggest challenge these retail giants will face is the inevitable clash between their core businesses and the huge investments they will need to make to invade healthcare's multitrillion-dollar industry. All companies, regardless of the industry, struggle with the challenge of trying to preserve what makes them successful today while pursuing that which has the potential to make them even more successful in the future. Amazon, CVS, and Walmart are all confronting this reality. And yet, you don't become the largest pharmacy company (CVS), largest online retailer (Amazon), or largest company, period, (Walmart) by chance or dumb luck.

What's more, most of the negative analyses concerning the retail giants ignore two things about the past healthcare failures of these companies. First, part of innovation is making errors and course correcting. The CEOs of these retail giants are comfortable with that reality. Be it drone deliveries or the Fire phone, Amazon's leaders seem unfazed by these types of mistakes. Second, these businesses have tens of billions of dollars on their balance sheets. A few misspent millions would be a rounding error for the world's largest retailers—a financial point of fact that not even the nation's largest health insurers can claim.

The retail giants aren't investing billions in healthcare because it is the "right thing to do." But that doesn't mean patients will suffer if the retailers win. On the contrary, higher quality with excellent access at affordable costs is a winning retail strategy, and it's also something that patients desire. What remains uncertain is whether a medical world dominated by the retail giants will be positive for physicians and other healthcare providers or even more problematic than today.

In this struggle for dominance, one thing is certain: to win at healthcare, CVS, Amazon, and Walmart can't be niche players in a narrow part of the healthcare ecosystem. For this reason, their recent healthcare acquisitions and partnerships should be seen merely as opening moves in a long game that will play out over the next decade. Eventually, they'll need to offer a full suite of healthcare services to Medicare enrollees, self-funded businesses, and ultimately every American.

Whether their current momentum will push these giants forward or the countervailing forces will push them back, only time will tell. What's clear is that the battle has begun. If doctors and traditional healthcare leaders want to defend their turf, they'll need to act quickly and learn to play by a whole new set of rules.

PART THREE | CHAPTER FOURTEEN

BREAKING THE RULES

At a leading academic hospital in greater New York, a 35-year-old singer named John has just undergone complex neck surgery. The operation went flawlessly, and the anesthesiologist has just extubated him (removed the breathing tube). But for some reason, John is having trouble breathing. The attending physician along with the chief resident feed a scope down the patient's throat to take a look. Both are shocked to see his vocal cords are nearly touching, restricting airflow and creating a potentially deadly crisis. They're confident they didn't damage any of the nerves to the larynx during surgery, which might've produced this result. And because neither physician has encountered this type of problem before, both are stumped.

Thankfully, it's 2024, and there's generative AI for that. Without delay, the senior resident reaches into her pocket, pulls out her iPhone and, with a few taps on ChatGPT, finds a case report identical to John's. Reading it, both doctors realize they haven't made a technical error after all. The case report reveals that, occasionally, the local anesthetic used during the procedure can spread beyond the operative area, temporarily impairing the vocal cord muscles. This reassurance proves correct when, just like the patient in the report, John's breathing normalizes within half an hour, readying him for discharge.

Without immediate access to this rare insight, John's doctors would have faced dire choices, including re-intubation and potential ICU admission. Failing to secure an airway could have led to an emergency tracheotomy, jeopardizing John's music career. While a traditional online search might've eventually unearthed the crucial case report,

ChatGPT's quick, intuitive interface provided the lifesaving information swiftly, showcasing the critical impact of on-the-spot expertise in emergency medical scenarios.

John's story shows how today's technology can help doctors prevent mistakes and provide better care. I've heard dozens of clinicians talk about how generative AI has helped them in various ways. In their offices, during hospital rounds, and in surgeries, physicians are using generative AI to improve their decisions, making sure they apply the most up-to-date medical information and optimal clinical recommendations to the patients they treat. This use of GenAI doesn't take away from what these doctors learned in school. Instead, it builds on that foundation.

Despite the great technological leaps made in recent years, medical education has been slow to adapt. Historically, medical schools and residency programs put a premium on the ability of applicants and trainees to memorize vast amounts of detailed information, with entrance and licensing exams designed to test this capacity. In the past, this almost singular emphasis on memorization made sense—without the internet or smartphones, a doctor might have needed to carry a 50-pound backpack filled with textbooks and medical journals to access the breadth of information necessary for superior care.

The technological landscape has shifted so significantly in medicine that mobile technologies equipped with ChatGPT now provide doctors with instant access to comprehensive, evidence-based medical information. The old era, where doctors relied heavily on their ability to recall medical facts, is transitioning to a new one. We are approaching a time when the ability to access and apply the best available medical knowledge accurately becomes more important than memory alone. In this era, effective communication with patients and staff also takes on heightened significance.

Yet, despite this technological revolution, academic institutions continue to prioritize traditional memorization skills instead of teaching students how to effectively use these new tools in their daily medical practice. Why is this? The answer has to do with the culture of medicine, which is—among many things—a collection of "rules."

More specifically, the culture of medicine comprises many *unwritten rules*, which dictate the "right way" to act. These rules, which influence clinician behavior, aren't taught in textbooks or lecture halls. They are observed and subconsciously absorbed by medical students and residents while trying to learn the ropes and earn the respect of physician leaders. Once absorbed, newly trained physicians carry these rules with them throughout their careers and eagerly pass them along to the next generation, ensuring their survival long past their utility.

These rules help explain why medical practice has been so slow to change. Indeed, most of healthcare's unwritten rules were established long ago, prior to 21st-century advances in science, technology, and clinical practice. And because many of them are now outdated, they obstruct clinical excellence. Unless broken, they will hold our nation back from reaching its full potential in Healthcare 4.0.

Tomorrow's patients will benefit most from healthcare professionals who can (a) understand and apply generative AI to discern the best, science-based approaches to diagnosis and treatment, (b) help patients use these modern technologies to access reliable information and monitor their own health and, (c) use office and telehealth visits to improve people's overall health.

The reality is that ChatGPT can already access and analyze a vast amount of information, surpassing the capacity of any single human. With regular updates and the ability to process multimodal information—from printed text to electronic healthcare records, bedside monitors, and the latest findings presented at national healthcare conferences—generative AI will redefine the skills doctors need to excel in medical care.

If medical professionals want to orchestrate meaningful change and lead the success of Healthcare 4.0, they can't simply bend the unwritten rules, tinker at the edges, or make small tweaks here and there. The full potential of generative AI hinges on the leadership within the medical community to boldly steer colleagues away from antiquated conventions that hold medicine back. Academic institutions must also embrace this shift, updating old educational paradigms to better equip future healthcare providers with the skills needed for this new era.

In Healthcare 4.0, the traditional emphasis on rote memorization must give way to a broader set of priorities, including the ability to leverage AI for enhanced patient care, the adoption of innovative practices, and a commitment to patient empowerment. Effective leadership will be crucial as practitioners navigate the transition from old methodologies to those more suited to the current landscape. Should the established medical field falter in this leadership role, retail behemoths and other newcomers stand ready to lead the charge. Here are a few of the other rules that will need to be broken:

1. Breaking the Rules That Prevent Integration

In most professions, hierarchy is determined by the level of influence and impact individuals have. Let's return to pro football for an example.

Although nothing in the rulebook grants relative status or authority to certain players, everyone knows the starting quarterback is the most valuable member of any team. That's because no other player can do more to win (or lose) a game.

The same rationale doesn't hold in medicine, and this lack of a logical pecking order stands in the way of delivering highly coordinated, well-integrated medical care. If saving a life is the most valuable thing a doctor can do, then surely the physicians who save the most lives should garner the most esteem. Instead, the relative rank of specialties is decided by this unwritten and outdated rule: "Doctors achieve high status by doing what seems impossible."

Throughout history, desperate patients have come to doctors hoping for a miracle. Physicians responded with incredible acts of healing—at times appearing to possess supernatural powers that defy known science. Doing the impossible not only elevates the overall prestige of the medical profession, it's also the overriding criterion for ranking people *within* it.

This explains why, for most of the last century, primary-care (internal medicine) doctors were held in the highest esteem. Their superpower, which set them apart from colleagues, was the ability to unravel medical mysteries. When cardiologists, pulmonologists, or orthopedists couldn't diagnose an ailment, they turned to primary care for expertise. Time and again, these brilliant diagnosticians did the impossible. However, the unwritten rule—the one that enshrined primary care in the 20th century—is the same rule that sent the specialty crashing down in the 21st.

Healthcare 1.0 brought with it an eruption of medical innovation. This period introduced the widespread use of MRIs and CT scanners, along with improvements in the quality of ultrasounds. These tools digitized diagnosis and radically improved medical practice. But they also turned a renowned skill of primary-care doctors into an average and unremarkable ability.

Meanwhile, surgeons and interventional subspecialists had embarked on a period of relentless innovation—boosting their status in medicine by doing what was once thought impossible.

Orthopedists, whose job in the previous century was to reset and cast broken bones, could now replace hip and knee joints with space-age implants. Ophthalmologists, who historically wrote prescriptions for eyeglasses, invented a way to restore the vision of patients with cataracts by removing the opaque lens and replacing it with a clear, artificial substitute. And incredibly, interventional cardiologists could now reverse myocardial infarctions by passing catheters into the heart, unblocking the occluded blood vessels.

These unbelievable advancements flipped the healthcare hierarchy on its head. Specialists were now seen as heroes, capable of impossible feats, while primary-care physicians were demoted in both status and pay.

And yet, if medicine were a meritocracy, the relative order in the medical profession today would make no sense at all. Research consistently shows that the most effective way to save lives isn't through complex surgeries or procedures, but by preventing chronic diseases and their life-threatening complications like heart attacks, strokes, systemic infections, and cancers. Yet, paradoxically, specialists who perform these high-stakes interventions are often elevated in status and compensation, earning two to three times more than primary-care physicians who are central to disease prevention and management.

This discrepancy in the healthcare hierarchy is at odds with the modern landscape of medical challenges. Chronic illnesses now account for seven in 10 American deaths and their prevalence is rising across the US. In this context, the interventions of specialists, while occasionally lifesaving, have a relatively minor impact on overall mortality compared to the potential gains from effective chronic-disease prevention and management. Consider the results of a study by Harvard and Stanford researchers in 2019. The team found that adding 10 primary-care doctors to a population of 100,000 people increases average life expectancy two and a half times more than adding 10 specialists.

In today's medical world, the complexity and multiplicity of chronic diseases call for a collaborative approach to healthcare, one that transcends the archetype of the singular heroic doctor. Teams of physicians working together offer the best chance for comprehensive care, with primary-care physicians ideally positioned to coordinate these efforts and lead the way. Yet, this collaborative model is hindered by an outdated hierarchy that undervalues primary care. For a true transformation in healthcare that prioritizes patient outcomes, this entrenched rule on status must be broken, recognizing the critical role of primary care in a modern, effective healthcare system.

Of course, in any profession, those with power and privilege are slow to cede either. But hierarchical change—and the integration of care—is possible.

To explain, let's return to the football analogy. There was a period when offensive linemen, much like today's primary-care physicians, were undervalued. However, smart football coaches eventually recognized the critical role of the left tackle in protecting the quarterback's blindside and preventing season-ending injuries. This shift in strategy elevated the importance and compensation of offensive tackles, making them some of the highest-drafted and highest-paid players in the NFL—after quarterbacks, of course.

Like the left tackle's duties on the football field, primary-care physicians play a similarly protective and preventive role in healthcare. They work tirelessly to maintain patient health and preempt medical complications before they spiral into emergencies. Yet, much like the unheralded lineman who executes crucial blocks unseen by most spectators, the contributions of primary-care physicians often go unnoticed. Just as the sport eventually recognized the value of the lineman, it is time US healthcare acknowledges and rewards the indispensable role of primary care in maintaining the health of patients and the stability of the entire system.

2. Breaking the Rules That Prevent Capitation

As previous chapters explained, patient problems have evolved greatly over time. They went from mostly acute and unexpected in the 20th century to predominantly chronic (heart disease, arthritis, diabetes, asthma, and so on) in this one. And as medical problems became more complicated, healthcare costs soared.

With the rise of powerful, for-profit insurance companies over the past two decades, doctors have been driven to see more and more patients per day—spending up to half of those visits on the computer for billing and claims documentation purposes. As a result, the relationship between patients and doctors has changed dramatically, and not for the better.

Amid these ups and downs, one aspect of healthcare has remained the same: the way we pay physicians. As it was in the last century, doctors still get paid quid pro quo. That is, they provide a service, submit a bill, receive a check, and repeat. These kinds of transactional payments are the basis for nearly all financial interactions in the United States. A seller provides a good or service in exchange for payment. This is how we hire piano teachers, rent apartments, and procure Girl Scout cookies. And it's also how we pay for 95 percent of all physician visits today.

Paying transactionally for healthcare made sense in simpler times when doctors could deliver only a fraction of the "products" and "services" they provide today. Let's consider surgery as an example.

In the 20th century, surgeons often had to make decisions with less information than we have today. Limited by the diagnostic tools of the time, it was incredibly difficult to differentiate between conditions like an inflamed appendix, which requires emergency surgery, and viral gastroenteritis, which usually gets better on its own. Given that the consequences of not treating a potentially ruptured appendix were far more severe than those of unnecessary exploratory surgery, surgeons frequently opted to operate in uncertain cases. As a result, even the most skilled surgeons found that in 15 percent of appendectomies, the removed appendix wasn't diseased. Since then, medical technology has advanced significantly. Now, we have better diagnostic tools that make it easier to determine whether a patient needs an appendectomy. Despite these technological advancements, the payment system has not fully evolved to reflect this progress. For instance, surgeons are compensated equally for an unnecessary appendectomy as they are for a lifesaving one.

Another example is the use of cardiac stents. The nonprofit Lown Institute found that one in five cardiac stents placed in American patients is unnecessary. Yet, the cardiologist performing this procedure gets paid the same amount, whether the stent was indicated or not. This mismatch—between the services that generate income and the services that prove best for recipients—leads to unnecessary procedures, increased healthcare costs, and greater risks to patients.

Researchers and policy experts point out that 25 percent of the $4 trillion spent on American healthcare each year is wasted (much of it on unnecessary or ineffective treatments). But excessive costs aren't the only complication of the traditional fee-for-service payment methodology. What's often overlooked are the ways that beneficial outcomes *aren't* achieved.

Fee-for-service not only overvalues intervention (e.g., surgery) but it also undervalues prevention (the avoidance of chronic disease and the life-threating complications they produce).

Under the current medical payment methodology, cardiologists are paid vastly more to perform an angioplasty than prevent a patient's heart attack in the first place. Similarly, surgeons are viewed as heroic when they transplant a kidney or lung, but little attention is paid to the errors of omission in medical care that allowed the organ to fail in the first place. This approach doesn't make sense either from the perspective of what is best for patients or for the health of our nation.

Herein lies the transactional payment problem: how do you pay someone appropriately for something that *didn't* happen (like a heart attack or a stroke)? In a fee-for-service reimbursement system, a primary-care doctor—working hard to help patients avoid these high-priced, life-threatening complications from chronic disease—has to file an insurance claim for each step along the way. To help just one patient effectively manage or prevent even one chronic disease, a physician may be required to submit dozens of claims, each paying the doctor relatively little. It should come as no surprise then that physicians fail to adequately control hypertension, screen for cancer, or achieve an acceptable glucose level in patients with diabetes. When you consider that 133 million Americans suffer from at least one chronic illness, it's clear that continuing to pay doctors transactionally is a costly error.

As the volume of procedures went up over the past two decades, insurers sought to reduce healthcare costs by lowering payments to doctors and implementing strict prior-authorization requirements. In a transactional payment model, these are just about the only tools an insurer has to curb medical spending and dial back unnecessary (as well as necessary) services. In response to ratcheted down payments, doctors have been forced to see more patients per day to maintain their incomes. And on top of that, they must invest several hours each day to obtain authorization and complete the required paperwork to do what they know to be best and be paid for it. As a result, they are frustrated and exhausted, suffering increased levels of burnout that leave them feeling robbed of the professional fulfillment they seek and deserve.

Transactional payments also harm the doctor-patient relationship. In a 2019 survey, physicians said that gratitude from, and relationships with, patients were the most rewarding aspects of medical practice. And yet, 87 percent of doctors say that patients trust them less now than a decade ago. Many factors contribute to the erosion of the doctor-patient relationship, but more than half of physicians (56 percent) point to healthcare costs as the primary cause of patient dissatisfaction. Increasingly, these financial frustrations spill over into the exam room.

Once again, healthcare's transactional payment model fuels the problem. Whenever the number and complexity of services dictate the payment amount—be it in medicine or car repair or home remodeling—the recipient of the service fears the provider may be trying to "upsell" them. For patients and doctors alike, this fear proves unhealthy, shredding the very fabric of their relationship.

Both the federal government and private insurance companies have tried to fix the problems of physician reimbursement with "pay for value" and "pay for performance" incentives. These programs are well intentioned, but they simply replace one form of transactional payment with another. Using these methodologies, payment depends on whether doctors order a preventive service or give advice, but not whether their efforts make any positive difference in the patient's health.

Instead of a quid pro quo payment methodology, American medicine needs to "break the rules" with a relationship-based reimbursement model. Capitation at the delivery system level (payments made directly to doctors and hospitals) would solve this problem.

But, of course, breaking a centuries-old rule of healthcare payments won't be easy. And it is unlikely to be accomplished overnight. A solid starting point would be for the Centers for Medicare & Medicaid Services to shift primary-care payments in the Medicare program in a way that allows physicians and patients to form "healthier" relationships. Here's how a *transformational*, relationship-based reimbursement system might be implemented as a first step.

- Medicare enrollees would select a primary-care doctor as their accountable physician.
- CMS would then pay that physician a single upfront sum to provide a year's worth of primary care to these patients (instead of a payment after each medical service).
- The doctor's base compensation would depend on (a) the number of Medicare enrollees they care for and (b) the complexity of each patient's current medical problems, which helps to forecast the amount of direct medical care they'll need.
- Each primary-care physician would be eligible for added payments, depending on the patient's experience. At the end of the year, enrollees would answer a series of questions about the impact their physician had over the previous 12 months: Did the doctor help you live a healthier life? Did the doctor help you make good medical decisions? Do you value your relationship? Do you trust your doctor's recommendations?

This transformational payment model would lead to greater professional satisfaction because doctors would no longer be paid on a "piecemeal" basis and would spend far less time on paperwork. And in place of these dissatisfying bureaucratic tasks, physicians would have more time to help patients prevent and manage their acute and chronic diseases. Further, this type of transformational payment would shift the incentives from what a doctor does to the impact a doctor has on the patient. Rather than evaluating physicians on a litany of individual actions and clinical metrics, the transformational model rewards physicians for the positive impact they have on the total health of their patients. That approach would save lives and resonate with the reason people choose to become doctors in the first place.

If our country can't break the unwritten rule for how doctors are paid, America's healthcare problems will continue to get worse.

3. Breaking the Rule That Prevents Patient-Empowering Tech

Only one US industry has failed to use information technology to cut costs, increase access to products and services, and improve quality. That's healthcare. Generative AI, combined with other modern technologies, will drive performance in healthcare as it has in manufacturing, retail, and finance—but only if doctors and device manufacturers break another long-held rule.

That unwritten and rarely acknowledged rule? The only technological tools worth using are those that benefit clinicians.

An example of this rule, and the problems it creates, is the operative robot. These multimillion-dollar machines look like space-aged command centers with doctors sitting in the captain's chair, directing the movements of several large robotic arms. It's easy to see the appeal: these machines are incredibly cool and the surgeons who use them are seen as rock stars on the cutting edge of medical practice. Medical journals overflow with descriptions of new and interesting applications for these technologies. It's therefore no surprise that the surgical robotics market is projected to grow by 42 percent annually over the next decade.

But there's a problem: independent research from 39 clinical studies has determined that robot-assisted surgeries have, at best, only minimal clinical advantages over other approaches, and most often none. They have so far failed to extend life expectancy or significantly reduce surgical complications. In fact, they take more operative time and prove far more expensive for patients than traditional procedures. Looking objectively at the impact this technology has on patients, the operative robot is a dud. But for the physicians using it and for the hospitals that purchase it, the machine is a financial megahit.

On the other side of this outdated rule, there are technologies like the electronic health record introduced at the start of Healthcare 2.0. This tool should have ensured that clinicians have comprehensive data on patients and information on evidence-based best practices at all times. And it should have produced major improvements in clinical outcomes. Instead, it has become a symbol of what's wrong with tech in medicine. Rather than simplifying medical care delivery, EHR systems are cumbersome and clunky, and they sit (literally) between doctors and patients. Their primary function isn't to improve clinical outcomes. It is to increase billing and revenue generation for providers. Year after year, the *Medical Economics* survey of "things ruining medicine for physicians" rates EHR usability at or near the top of the list.

The contrast between the high-tech allure of operative robots and the cumbersome reality of EHR systems exemplifies this rule's detrimental impact. While robots are embraced for their futuristic appeal and revenue potential, despite minimal patient benefits, EHRs, which could revolutionize patient care by providing comprehensive, accessible data, became burdensome financial tools.

To transform healthcare, the new "rule" must prioritize technologies that not only enhance patient empowerment but also amplify the collaborative dynamic between patients and their physicians.

Take generative AI. Its potential to revolutionize healthcare isn't in question—we know it could significantly reduce mortality rates annually. Yet, the crux of its success hinges on a symbiotic relationship between healthcare providers and patients. While advanced versions of ChatGPT might equip patients with critical insights, such as the necessity for medication adjustments or surgical interventions, these recommendations still necessitate the expertise and hands-on involvement of a medical professional for actual implementation. For healthcare to evolve toward higher quality, increased accessibility, and greater affordability, while simultaneously alleviating physician burnout, a radical departure from traditional practices is essential.

We need a new criterion for appraising technological advancements in healthcare—one that focuses on patient-centric outcomes over physician-centric benefits. This rule shift will compel clinicians to view and value technology through the prism of patient impact, ensuring that innovations genuinely serve those they are meant to heal.

Overcoming Our Fears of Breaking the Rules

Transitioning to a healthcare system augmented by generative AI is not just about making technological upgrades. It's a paradigm shift in how we approach health and wellness. This change requires us to confront and dismantle long-standing rules and norms that have shaped the medical profession for decades.

In 1977, Ken Olsen, then CEO of Digital Equipment Corporation—a leading computer company of its time—reputedly declared that there was no reason for American families to have a computer in their homes.

This sentiment reflected the prevailing mindset of the day. It was based on a time when large, cumbersome mainframes dominated the computing field, and the idea of a home-based alternative seemed ridiculous. Had the industry failed to look forward, the widespread ownership of personal computers might never have materialized. Instead, most American households now own multiple computers and would find it almost impossible to maintain their lifestyle without one.

This historical shift in information technology—from mammoth mainframe computers to personal computers—mirrors the potential transformation of medicine in the era of Healthcare 4.0. As patients become empowered by technology, their demand for such capabilities will grow and more innovative solutions will arise. How quickly this desire will be fulfilled, and the magnitude of its impact, will depend on whether physicians encourage and support maximal patient expertise or resist sharing control.

Rather than viewing ChatGPT and other generative AI tools as threats to their status, clinicians should view them as opportunities to improve their lives and the lives of their patients. This synergy between technology and human expertise will produce a healthcare system that is more efficient, empathetic, and effective—assuming doctors support it.

For physicians, the advent of Healthcare 4.0 is not just a technological shift but a profound change in their professional identity. They are transitioning from being the sole keepers of medical wisdom to collaborative partners guiding patients on their health journey. This transformation, while initially challenging, holds the promise of returning a sense of control to both doctors and their patients, freeing them from the constraints of insurer-driven care while enhancing the patient care experience. Fundamentally, this shift highlights the true nature of medicine: the deep human connection and the art of healing.

Yet, this optimistic vision does not overlook the hurdles ahead. Issues such as privacy, security, and AI bias present ethical and legal challenges that will require careful consideration and proactive management. The risk of misinformation and the reliability of AI-generated guidance are concerns that will need ongoing attention and continuous refinement. These challenges, along with other apprehensions, will be the focus of part four.

PART FOUR
GENTLY

PART FOUR | CHAPTER FIFTEEN

ETHICS, PRIVACY, AND TRUST

Imagine yourself as the daring protagonist in a thrilling *Mission Impossible* scenario. Your mission, should you choose to accept it, has nothing to do with infiltrating secure vaults or chasing villains around the globe. Instead, you stand at the forefront of a healthcare revolution, armed with ChatGPT as your tool of choice. The risks are real, but so are the rewards.

Should you, brave patient, choose to embrace GenAI, you'll be stepping into a new realm of unprecedented medical care. You'll obtain the kind of personalized attention once exclusive to high-end retail and luxury hospitality. You'll enter a healthcare landscape where every medical professional you encounter is already intimately acquainted with your health history, genetic blueprint, and lifestyle choices. There'll be no need for repetitive recounts on your part. Envision it, a digital guardian by your hospital bedside, monitoring your well-being around the clock, warding off the specters of medical mishaps with an ever-watchful eye. In this brave new world, omnipresent AI technologies will become the custodians of your health, wielding a deep knowledge of your physiological infrastructure—far beyond any one doctor's comprehension.

As you stand ready to leap toward the future, apprehension stirs within. Unlike the dauntless Ethan Hunt, who confronts peril with unwavering resolve, the thought of entrusting such intimate aspects of your life to machines ignites a storm of anxiety and uncertainty in you. The shadowy possibilities of AI errors, privacy breaches, ethical dilemmas, security vulnerabilities, and skewed algorithms loom large.

The decision to embrace or eschew AI in healthcare is fraught with uncertainty. Americans will need to decide how to answer the high-stakes questions involved. Will they choose to embark on this mission, accepting the inherent risks for the promise of a transformed healthcare system? Or will caution tether them to the familiar, and compromised, clinical outcomes of traditional medicine?

***

A little more than a year before this book's publication, OpenAI launched its first publicly available generative AI system. The company's initial research on generative models began in 2016. And its very first version, the foundational GPT-1, launched in 2018 without public fanfare. At that time, OpenAI was known primarily within the research community and tech circles—a complete unknown to those outside the industry. Researchers and developers in the fields of artificial intelligence and machine learning used GPT-1 to explore capabilities in various language-processing tasks, but few individuals predicted how powerful it would become or the broad range of applications and user engagements that later models would achieve. Three years and 2.5 generations later, ChatGPT was released to the public, as part of a free research preview. By fall of 2023, more than 100 million people were using ChatGPT on a weekly basis.

As of this book's publication, ChatGPT has evolved beyond its initial 1,000 plugins to introduce custom "GPTs." These customizable features combine tailored instructions, expanded knowledge bases, and a blend of skills, enabling OpenAI's model to tap into external data sources, execute specialized tasks, and deliver responses that are most relevant to the context. A pivotal enhancement in early 2024 introduced a "memory" feature to ChatGPT, empowering the AI to recall previous interactions and utilize this information in subsequent conversations. These two advancements hold significant promise for healthcare applications.

With custom GPTs, patients will be able to input their medical data directly into the AI system. The memory feature will then allow ChatGPT to access and utilize this rich, personalized health information in future discussions. Looking ahead, this technology will enable physicians to tailor GPTs specifically for their patients, thereby enhancing the customization and personalization of medical care.

When asked about the potential for these updates to impact healthcare, ChatGPT replied: "The integration of custom GPTs and AI memory into healthcare systems represents a significant leap forward in personalized medicine. Custom GPTs enable healthcare professionals to tailor AI's responses and functionalities to meet the specific needs of their patients, thereby enhancing the precision of medical advice and interventions. Meanwhile, the introduction of memory allows for a more coherent and context-aware interaction between patients and AI, ensuring that each patient's medical history and unique health circumstances are considered in ongoing care. Together, these advancements promise to make healthcare more responsive, effective, and centered around the individual needs of each patient, marking a pivotal moment in the evolution of Healthcare 4.0."

Despite the massive future potential generative AI promises, doctors and patients remain ambivalent about its use in healthcare. A 2023 international GE survey revealed that only 26 percent of medical professionals in the United States think artificial intelligence can be trusted. Patients, meanwhile, are split. Nearly 70 percent of those surveyed by Deloitte's Center for Health Solutions believe generative AI is "very" or "extremely" reliable when it comes to healthcare. In fact, researchers found that one in five consumers who use ChatGPT have already relied on it to learn about their medical conditions. In contrast, a recent Pew poll found that 60 percent of American adults said they'd be "uncomfortable" with their doctor relying on artificial intelligence to diagnose their medical problems and provide treatment recommendations.

Having tested ChatGPT and dozens of other GenAI for more than a year now, I've seen these tools get continuously smarter, more reliable, and increasingly user friendly. And yet, even though the generative AI applications keep improving and drawing from an ever-larger corpus of knowledge, they continue to make mistakes. In writing this book, with ChatGPT as my coauthor, I witnessed a litany of both mind-boggling AI feats alongside inexplicable AI errors.

These generative AI systems still occasionally fail at basic math, make up sources and "hallucinate," providing confident yet factually incorrect responses. These tools stubbornly refuse instructions in some cases and, in others, maintain a strange people-pleasing quality, turning misleading or poorly constructed prompts (requests) into a string of gibberish, rather than prompting humans to improve their instructions. ChatGPT has no problem "ghosting" its users in the middle of a conversation, shutting down the chat with only an error message as apology.

ChatGPT, while powerful and revolutionary, has other limitations too, particularly in terms of currency. As of this book's publication, ChatGPT's corpus of knowledge is only current through April 2023, though ChatGPT can query Bing, Microsoft's internet search platform, for the most up-to-date information. Meanwhile, Google's generative AI product Gemini includes the totality of material available through the company's extensive websites, browsers, and knowledge graph, along with internally developed training data. While these approaches enhance the freshness of the information provided, they also introduce challenges: like distinguishing between valid scientific insights and potentially erroneous or misleading content, a concern we will explore in the following chapter. Moving forward, generative AI tools like ChatGPT will need to incorporate the latest scientific findings into their responses, necessitating regular updates and rigorous verification processes. This will help ensure the accuracy of the AI's knowledge base while also presenting challenges in discerning genuine scientific insights from those influenced by political or questionable motives.

But given the current constraints, it's prudent to exercise caution when considering medical advice from ChatGPT. At this stage, GPT-4 represents the dawn of Healthcare 4.0—a period of experimentation and refinement. We're far from understanding all the ways generative AI will ultimately shape healthcare. Yet, looking ahead five years, with technology projected to be 30 times more potent, the possibilities for diagnosis, disease management, and patient empowerment are immense and promising.

Throughout history, people have been hesitant to embrace new technology, meeting the majority of innovations with skepticism and concerns over reliability. Yet, time and again, as technologies prove their worth, suspicion turns to astonishment. We look back, wondering how we ever doubted these advancements that have become so integral to our lives.

Take the mercury thermometer as an example. After its invention in 1714, it took another 100 years for Daniel Fahrenheit's groundbreaking tool to become standard in medical practice. This lag persisted despite decades of scientific proof that it was more accurate in measuring temperature and assessing fever than doctors who relied on skin-to-skin touch. Today, the thought of assessing a fever without a thermometer is inconceivable.

Consider the introduction of the telephone, too. Invented by Alexander Graham Bell in 1876, the earliest phones faced widespread doubt and slow adoption. People accustomed to face-to-face conversations and handwritten correspondence found the idea of speaking to someone not physically present unsettling. It took years for society to grasp its potential and integrate it into daily life. Today, the thought of a world without smartphones—the telephone's modern descendants—is unimaginable.

Even ATMs gave bank customers pause in the 1970s, fearing the machines would eat their cards and mishandle their money. Indeed, cashpoint errors were common at first, fueling these concerns. However, as banks refined the technology and improved reliability, customer apprehension faded from consciousness. And now, we're moving toward a future where virtual deposits are becoming the norm, making in-person and ATM transactions increasingly obsolete.

This progressive comfort with technology is known as *habituation*. And when it comes to using generative AI in medicine, habituating won't take patients and doctors 100 years or even a decade. But it will likely follow a similar arc: beginning with skepticism, fears, and reports of failure, followed by research trials, specific use cases, and ever more examples of superiority. This trajectory will ultimately result in widespread use and broad acceptance.

Given the tremendous expertise of the software developers in OpenAI—and more than 2 million developers currently building on the company's API—along with top minds and tech talent at Google, Amazon, Microsoft, and most Fortune 500 firms, we can expect that today's application errors will diminish significantly in the near future.

But before our nation places its health and trust in the hands of generative AI, OpenAI and its competitors will need to prove themselves worthy of our acceptance by eliminating, or at least acknowledging, our fears. This section of the book examines some of the thorniest issues presented by generative AI in the early days of Healthcare 4.0.

Fear 1: Security

Banks, government bodies, and healthcare companies alike house sensitive information in large databases and, therefore, face major security threats. That's especially true now, as more and more data move to the cloud (the internet-based servers on which these large databases run). Research shows nine in 10 Americans are worried hackers will access their personal or financial information and use it for nefarious purposes. Although concerns about internet and cloud security are valid, I question whether generative AI will *increase* people's personal risk of future cyberattacks.

For perspective—and contrary to what patients might assume—a solo doctor's office is one of the least secure places to house personal medical data today. Lone physician practices lack the financial and technological resources to install top-of-the-line network security tools, which therefore make patient data extremely vulnerable. The only reason these offices are not a frequent target of cybercriminal hacking is that large data systems—containing hundreds of thousands or even millions of patient records—are much more valuable.

Ironically, the thing that makes medical records safer inside your local doctor's office is the same thing that makes the medical-record system ineffective as a whole. Unless your doctor belongs to a large medical group, your personal health record isn't likely to be connected (or available) to other physician offices or surrounding hospitals. Though government health officials have tried for decades to incentivize secure patient-record sharing (interoperability), very few providers today can access a "comprehensive" medical-record system. As a result, even when clinicians in the community use the same digital record-keeping platform, they can't quickly obtain the information needed to provide optimal medical care to each patient.

This isn't just ineffective, it's also dangerous. If you end up in the ER late at night when your doctor's office is closed, the emergency physician on staff can't look up your medical history, current prescriptions, recent diagnostic tests, or the other vital information needed to provide you with the best care possible.

As such, security in medicine walks a fine line. As patients, we want our medical data to be safely off-limits to malicious hackers. But we also need that information to be readily available wherever we go for care, regardless of the time of day or day of the week.

Generative AI faces the same security threats as electronic health records and our bank information, but no more. Meaning, there's nothing specific to the creation or operation of these AI tools that will increase people's cybersecurity risks. In the same way that large financial institutions and EHR companies store vast quantities of digitized information behind firewalls that are difficult to penetrate, we can assume that ChatGPT (and the generative AI systems developed by Google and others) will maintain at least equal safeguards. It is in their reputational and economic interests to do so.

Fear 2: Privacy

Although large IT companies work hard to maximize data security, some of their business models depend on compromising user privacy. For example, a congressperson once asked Mark Zuckerberg how Facebook survives as a business without charging user fees. Without blinking, the founder, chair, and CEO of Meta responded, "By advertising."

Foundational to Meta's advertising model is the sale of user data to third parties. For decades, the people who use social media sites and search engines have been making a de facto trade: handing over their personal information to advertisers in exchange for free access to the platforms.

In medicine, it's illegal to extract and disclose data from individual medical records. But that doesn't guarantee total patient privacy. Recently, news reports exposed how hospitals and pharmacies engage in online data sharing with third parties—without explicit permission from patients. Moreover, when people search their symptoms on the internet, click on links, or make online purchases to treat health problems, that information has been used by companies to target ads. It is why people receive coupons for diapers within days of learning they're pregnant.

Patients may face similar privacy risks with generative AI companies. But as with security, there's nothing specific to generative AI that magnifies user privacy risks. Moreover, ChatGPT generates enough income through a subscription model that it doesn't need to involve third party advertisers, at least not yet. Finally, laws like HIPAA in the United States provide guidelines for the protection of patient data. Hopefully, as AI technology evolves, so will these regulations.

Fear 3: Bias
Unlike in the areas of security and privacy, where Pew survey respondents indicated high levels of concern, most patients predict that generative AI will be less medically biased in the future (51 percent), not more biased (15 percent).

However, not all forms of AI have the same level of neutrality. Researchers continue to identify biases in both the rule-based and narrow AI tools used in medicine today. In several cases, these IT applications have been shown to exacerbate existing healthcare inequities (gaps in the quality of care based on gender, race, ethnicity, income, etc.).

In one infamous example, a study published in *Science* found that a predictive healthcare algorithm had discriminated against Black patients. The tool, created by Optum (the tech branch of UnitedHealth Group), was designed to identify high-risk patients with poorly treated chronic diseases, thereby helping the company augment medical resources for those who'd benefit most. But there was a glitch in the algorithm, according to researchers. Rather than ranking the needs of patients based on the severity or complexity of their illnesses, the algorithm relied on a surrogate measure: the cost of each patient's past treatments. It assumed that more spending on medical services equated to greater need for medical services.

The problem with that approach is that Black patients across the country receive $1,800 less medical care each year than white patients with the same disease burden. And as a result, Black patients were significantly underrepresented in the group selected by Optum for additional medical services.

When the researchers went back and re-ranked patients by the severity of their illnesses (rather than the cost of care), the percentage of Black patients who should have been enrolled in specialized care programs jumped from 17.7 percent to 46.5 percent. Once the error was discovered, Optum's now-notorious algorithm became the subject of intense media scrutiny, resulting in widespread outrage throughout the scientific community.

News coverage of the controversy left no doubt about who (or, rather, what) was to blame. "US Hospital Algorithm Discriminates Against Black Patients," read a *British Medical Journal* headline. "Racial Bias Found In A Major Healthcare Risk Algorithm," said *Scientific American*. "Millions Of Black People Affected By Racial Bias In Healthcare Algorithms," noted *Nature*.

While media headlines were quick to point the finger at the AI tool, the root of the problem lay with implicit human bias, not with the technology itself. It wasn't the algorithm that discriminated against Black patients. It was the result of physicians subconsciously providing Black patients with insufficient and inequitable treatment. In other words, the biased outcomes stemmed from human actions and decisions, not from a programming error.

The reality is that the bias in question happened in the medical offices and hospitals where patients were treated, long before the computer work began. If Black patients had received equivalent medical care to white patients over the preceding years, the AI application would have been accurate in its conclusions and free of bias.

For decades, however, American medical practice has enabled and perpetuated discrimination against patients of color, providing them with suboptimal care.

For example, US doctors recommend breast reconstruction for Black patients following mastectomy less often than for white patients. They prescribe less pain medication to Black and Hispanic patients than white individuals after surgery. And early in the pandemic, when Black individuals were twice as likely to die from COVID-19, physicians tested Black patients for the virus only half as often as white patients with identical symptoms.

Contrary to rule-based and narrow AI, generative AI has the potential to reduce, rather than increase, the prevalence of bias in medicine. That's because it includes a much broader range of inputs than the narrow AI applications developed for specific medical functions (like reading mammograms, managing diabetes, or figuring out which patients would benefit the most from added resources). In contrast to these other types of AI, generative AI has been constructed to answer a nearly infinite number of questions and perform an unlimited number of functions.

To facilitate that ability, the applications have been pre-trained using vast data sets—ones that may unintentionally include biases in patient care but also include evidenced-based research on the existence and dangers of bias in medicine. So, when physicians "forget" to offer breast reconstruction, prescribe adequate pain medication, or order a necessary laboratory test for Black or Hispanic patients, ChatGPT can question the doctor's decisions. In this way, it will bend the arc of care delivery away from medical bias and toward a more equitable form of healthcare treatment for all.

Because generative AI encompasses a broader spectrum of data, including vast amounts of medical literature that cover both clinical best practices *and* the sociocultural aspects of medicine, this inclusivity of data will allow ChatGPT to train itself to detect bias in healthcare. Thus, when there's a discrepancy in care—such as the under-prescription of pain medication to minority patients—generative AI will be able to prompt healthcare providers to reconsider their decisions; providing data-driven recommendations that align with best practices for all patient demographics. This function will act as a counterweight to human errors, nudging the healthcare system toward fairness and equality for all patients, regardless of their background.

Fear 4: Reliability
Unlike objective science, which derives from data, trust is subjective. As the Optum study in *Science* showed, humans tend to blame technology harshly when it fails to perform as desired or expected—much harsher than when people, themselves, make even graver errors.

As evidence, consider how little attention is paid to the roughly 40,000 traffic deaths on US roadways that humans cause each year. Given the high death toll, you might think drivers would be eager to embrace driverless vehicles. But, according to University of Michigan researchers, that's not remotely true.

"For consumers to accept driverless vehicles … tests will need to prove with 80 percent confidence that they're 90 percent safer than human drivers," read the report.

Going by these numbers, humans would *not* embrace self-driving cars if they *only* prevented 20,000 or 30,000 deaths annually. To be considered safe enough to replace humans, driverless cars would need to save more than 35,000 lives each year. In practical terms, this means autonomous vehicles must prevent nearly all the deaths currently attributed to human mistakes on the road, not just a fraction, to overcome public skepticism and be deemed a viable replacement.

The now-familiar motif of "man vs. machine" has been around since the industrial revolution, dating back to the Luddite Rebellion of the early 1800s wherein English textile workers destroyed mechanical looms that threatened to automate their jobs. For modern-day interpretations of this phobia, see *2001: A Space Odyssey* or *West World*.

In healthcare, an example of our pro-human bias manifests in how little attention we pay to avoidable medical errors and misdiagnoses, which kill hundreds of thousands of Americans each year. Were ChatGPT responsible for causing even a single medical death in 2024, it would dominate news coverage—just as a Tesla Model 3 did in February when the full-self-driving vehicle "barreled into a tree and exploded in flames, killing … a Tesla employee and devoted fan of CEO Elon Musk," according to the Washington Post.

In medicine, the death toll from preventable medical mistakes is akin to six large passenger jets crashing every day of the year with no survivors. And yet, most people never worry about or even contemplate this massive medical failure.

Human mistakes in healthcare are the third-leading cause of death in the United States (behind heart disease and cancer). Prior to the COVID-19 pandemic, a pair of independent studies found that 50 to 63 percent of US women who get regular mammograms over 10 years will receive at least one "false-positive" interpretation, which leads to additional testing and unnecessary procedures.

In fact, one-third of the time, when two or more radiologists look at the same mammograms, they will disagree in their interpretation of the results. That means that a third of the time, one of the radiologists will be wrong. Presently, visual pattern recognition software, having been trained on thousands of images, is estimated to be 5 to 10 percent more accurate than mammographers, and the technology is continually improving.

The superiority of AI tools compared to humans extends far beyond mammography. Already, narrow AI solutions have been able to identify lung and breast cancer and diagnose pneumonia on chest X-rays just as reliably or even better than the best radiologists today. And they do so in a matter of seconds, allowing patients to rapidly know the results of their study.

The accuracy gap between humans and artificial intelligence is widening, too. As machines become more powerful and deep-learning approaches gain traction, they will continue to advance their diagnostic proficiency in radiology (CT, MRI, and mammography interpretation), pathology (microscopic and cytological diagnoses), dermatology (rash identification and pigmented lesion evaluation for potential melanoma), and ophthalmology (retinal vessel examination to predict the risk for diabetic retinopathy and cardiovascular disease).

AI applications can't yet make perfect diagnoses from visual images. But in cases where they're more accurate than radiologists, we should re-evaluate our confidence in humans and our distrust of technology.

The reality is that people trust humans far more than they trust machines, even when the data demonstrate they shouldn't. This discrepancy stems partly from our lack of understanding of AI technology, but a significant portion arises from apprehension about AI's future role. A clear example of this happened in 2023 when the Screen Writers' Guild and the union representing actors went on strike over the threat that generative AI posed to their professions and livelihoods. Of course, Hollywood isn't alone in this fear. Lawyers, teachers, consultants, writers, stockbrokers and, yes, even clinicians harbor the same types of concerns.

According to one study, artificial intelligence is set to take over 47 percent of the US employment market within 20 years. Though blue-collar jobs have long been in technology's crosshairs, doctors, nurses, and other health professionals are starting to feel the pressure, too. Without question, the role of the physician will change in the future. But it is unlikely generative AI will completely replace human-to-human relationships.

In fact, I'm optimistic that the doctor-patient relationship will become stronger in the future, assuming physicians choose to embrace rather than resist the inevitable progress of generative AI. And if they do, I'm confident the combination of human plus technology will not only produce superior clinical outcomes and more convenient access for patients but also lower costs by reducing chronic diseases, avoiding medical errors, and eliminating ineffective medical care.

The discussion about technology in healthcare frequently skirts the sensitive issue of AI taking over clinicians' roles. Pundits assert that AI will *supplement* rather than *supplant* doctors. I have a more nuanced outlook on this.

I believe that within five to 10 years, technologies like ChatGPT will be capable of performing approximately 20 percent of the tasks that doctors handle today. And with ChatGPT assuming responsibilities for monitoring chronic diseases, managing people's symptoms, and addressing patient inquiries about medication dosages for anticoagulants or insulin drugs, today's doctors will find themselves with more time in their day. Twenty percent more time each day translates to hundreds more hours per year. With added time, physicians will be able to engage more deeply with patients' concerns. Doctors can end their workdays with a greater sense of fulfillment, knowing they haven't compromised on care quality. And with their physicians less rushed, patients can receive more focused and personalized attention, allowing for a deeper exploration of their health concerns. This will lead to more accurate diagnoses, more thoughtful treatment plans, and a stronger doctor-patient relationship. Ultimately, patients will feel heard and valued and, therefore, will be more likely to adhere to the most up-to-date clinical recommendations and experience higher satisfaction with their care.

To prepare the profession and patients for these changes, medical schools will have to instruct students in the development and use of advanced AI systems. In parallel, the National Institutes of Health and other regulatory bodies will need to support the effort by comparing the clinical outcomes that clinician-plus-ChatGPT achieves versus doctors alone. I'm confident this analytic process will augment the trust people have in using this technology based on objective data, not human biases.

Generative AI: Healthcare Hero or Villain?
Trust is a funny thing. When we imagine a robot performing surgery or a computer program diagnosing a rare illness, it sounds overly futuristic—far from our present reality. But the entire history of innovation involves shifting progressively from the impossible to the possible to the day-to-day.

There was a time when the idea of continuously monitoring our own health metrics through a smartwatch—or controlling our home environment with voice commands connected to a smart speaker—would have seemed too complex or even risky. Yet, these technologies have become commonplace, seamlessly integrating into our daily routines. In the future, generative AI technology will play a similar role for patients when it comes to their medical care, simplifying and enhancing the way they manage their health—all with the same ease and convenience consumers have come to expect from financial and home automation tools.

What's unique about generative AI is the pace at which it is becoming more reliable and available. In fact, the greatest fear of many who are experts in generative AI isn't that it will fail to become incredibly powerful and capable of producing unimaginable outcomes. It is that it will be too powerful and pose an existential threat to human existence.

In one frequently cited study, AI researchers and other experts were asked: "What probability do you put on human inability to control future advanced AI systems causing human extinction?" The median answer was 10 percent. That's not nearly as threatening as, say, 50 percent, but it certainly not as comforting as zero.

***

The threat and the promise of AI strikes at the heart of our deepest fears and greatest hopes, a conflict that played out in late 2023 inside OpenAI. In the span of five white-knuckle days in November, Sam Altman, the head of Silicon Valley's most advanced generative AI company was fired by his board of directors, replaced by not one but two different candidates, hired to lead Microsoft's AI-research efforts and, finally, rehired back to his CEO position at OpenAI with a new board. A couple of weeks later, *TIME* selected him "CEO of the Year."

But Altman's saga is more than a tale of tech-industry intrigue. Many believe it came down to an existential question about the future of humanity. Contrary to media reports, I believe Altman and the now-disbanded board actually shared a common mission: to save humanity.

The problem was that the parties were 180 degrees apart when it came to defining how best to protect humankind. Altman's path to saving humanity involved racing forward as fast as possible. As CEO, he understood generative AI's potential to radically enhance productivity and alleviate threats like world hunger and climate change. By contrast, the board feared that breakneck AI development could spiral out of control, posing a threat to human existence. Rather than perceiving AGI (artificial general intelligence) as a savior, much of the board worried that a self-learning system might harm humanity.

This dichotomy pitted a CEO intent on changing the world ASAP against a board intent on proceeding at a cautious, incremental pace. Ultimately, I believe the biggest risk to humanity emanates from people misusing technology for nefarious purposes, not from the technology itself. Trust will be essential, but figuring out how to ensure that humans don't use technology to produce harm will be equally vital.

Putting the pieces together, while AI applications can't fully eliminate people's security, privacy, and bias fears—no matter how reliable it becomes—the risk to users should be no more than what people already experience. In contrast, the upside potential of this technology will be significantly greater than what exists today. With Healthcare 4.0 upon us, GenAI will provide opportunities to improve the health of patients, reduce the burnout of clinicians, and make medical care affordable. But before it can do that, there's another set of risks that will need to be addressed. The problem of human generated misinformation will be the next chapter's focus.

PART FOUR | CHAPTER SIXTEEN

MISINFORMATION AND MEDICAL CREDIBILITY

When it comes to security, privacy, and bias, the line between what's appropriate and deceptive is fairly clear cut and well-defined. Hacking into people's medical information is illegal and wrong. Selling an individual's medical data is rightly forbidden, but buying and trading aggregate user data is simply the price we pay for access to our digital world. And, of course, all of us would rather see less bias, not more, in the AI tools researchers use.

In contrast, the material in this chapter will prove more contentious, spotlighting the ambiguous divide between medical information and misinformation, between truth and deception in healthcare. Whereas most Americans agree on issues involving privacy breaches and biased algorithms, debates over misinformation play out on a complex battlefield. Day after day, polarizing perspectives and personal beliefs compete with scientific evidence, highlighting the tensions between our censorship concerns and our pursuit of scientific fact.

***

During the COVID-19 pandemic, the United States was engulfed in a silent battle over information dissemination. In an age already defined by "alternative facts," partisan news, and online echo chambers, clear divisions emerged regarding the control of public-facing medical information during the health crisis. Traditionally, public-health guidance was disseminated through doctor's offices and community health centers, with input from authoritative bodies like the Centers for Disease Control and Prevention and the U.S. Food and Drug Administration. However, the digital age saw this battleground swiftly move to the realm of social media, where varied and conflicting voices vied for influence.

Pinterest, the go-to social platform for kitchen makeovers and kitschy fashions, took a stand—blocking vaccine-related search terms on its platform in February 2019. The company explained that anti-vaccine content had run amok, contradicting evidence-based science and established research. While the search ban was only temporary, the effort was a notable departure from the long-held, unofficial policy of tech giants—most do everything in their power to *avoid* policing health content and conversations.

Under increased pressure, other digital platforms like Facebook explored ways to block discredited medical information and cut off revenue streams to users who posted anti-vaccine conspiracy theories—before eventually backing off. YouTube, for its part, disabled ads on "anti-vaxx" channels so that those users could not profit from advertising.

At the time, I applauded Pinterest for taking by far the biggest step toward shutting down posts that contained anti-vaccine recommendations. And I rooted, publicly, for other companies that committed to protecting visitors from false and dangerous health content.

However, I also recognized the challenge involved. Balancing the protection of patients from misinformation *without* limiting their access to essential medical updates was no easy task. Even reputable sources like the CDC and World Health Organization unintentionally shared inaccurate information during the pandemic.

Our nation continues to confront myriad issues involving free speech, access to reliable medical information, and "fake news," predicaments for which there are still no easy answers. And when it comes to curbing misinformation, generative AI presents a mixed bag in the eyes of many.

On one hand, ChatGPT can provide quick, accessible insights, potentially democratizing health knowledge and expertise. However, this same technology also harbors the potential to generate and amplify health misinformation. AI's ability to create convincing but inaccurate or misleading content can pose serious risks. For instance, AI-generated fake news articles, misleading health advice, "deep fake" videos of credible figures, or fabricated patient testimonials could easily circulate online, misleading patients and healthcare providers alike. Others fear that that echo chamber effect might extend to AI as sophisticated algorithms inadvertently push misleading health narratives more and more to susceptible individuals, reinforcing false beliefs and potentially dangerous behaviors.

On the other hand, generative AI tools like ChatGPT also offer a promising *solution* to the pervasive challenge of online health misinformation. Unlike conventional search engines that often prioritize engaging or polarizing content to drive ad revenue, potentially leading to the amplification of sensationalized or inaccurate medical advice, ChatGPT operates on a different principle. Its subscription-based model incentivizes the provision of accurate, balanced, and level-headed information, making it a potentially more reliable source for medical guidance. Moreover, the sophisticated algorithms of generative AI enable it to discern and prioritize high-quality information from reputable sources. By continuously updating its knowledge base with the latest peer-reviewed research and official health guidelines, ChatGPT can mitigate the risk of propagating misinformation.

Generative AI has the power and potential to replace traditional internet search tools that have for decades dispensed unreliable medical advice. Unlike search engines and sites that drive ad sales through "click-bait" headlines and pot stirring, ChatGPT's subscription model means the app does best when it produces more balanced, level-headed information. However as next-generation apps roll out, ChatGPT and its peers will be trained on a broader spectrum of internet sources for learning, which poses some of the same risks as search engines do (unintentionally disseminating misinformation from sources who appear credible).

Here are two steps generative AI companies could take to protect patients from misinformation in the era of Healthcare 4.0.

1. Fortify the Algorithms and Parameters

Back in 2011, Google launched its "Panda" algorithm update and, in so doing, began raising the bar on the quality of its search returns. Panda was a necessary reaction to clever web marketers who had been gaming Google's algorithms for years, stuffing web pages with "keywords" to boost their page ranking in searches. In its quest to improve the validity of content suggestions, the search giant revealed the kinds of questions that helped it discern good sources from bad. Questions like these served as guidance for anyone hoping to publish a high-ranking article: "Would you trust the information presented in this article?" and "Does this article have spelling, stylistic, or factual errors?" and "Is the article short, unsubstantial, or otherwise lacking in helpful specifics?"

Whether or not people noticed, the update worked—to an extent. Websites that used sneaky tricks like "keyword stuffing" to boost their search ratings suddenly stopped appearing in search engine results pages (or SERPs). What's more, Google refined Panda over and over again, releasing more than a dozen versions to stay ahead of spammers.

When it comes to generative AI, companies like OpenAI and Google could self-regulate to help avoid misinformation, insisting on transparency and integrity when it comes to the parameters ("rules") they use to select medical content.

As an example, they could program their tools to rely on information from "high impact journals," a commonly used measure of how many researchers and scientists refer to a particular published article. This is, in essence, a demonstration of professional recognition for the validity of the work. AI companies can and do create parameters during AI training that elevate sources perceived to be more reliable than others. To maximize transparency, AI companies could insist on revealing whether advice comes from reports published in a peer-reviewed journal, an accredited academic center, or data released by an agency like the FDA or part of an NIH grant. These companies could also indicate when data or recommendations may be vulnerable to conflicts of interest.

Most likely, the leading generative AI models will continue to provide more reliable information than can be found on the internet or social media for several reasons. First, as noted before, the financial model of

OpenAI doesn't rely on traffic volume, but instead on attracting users wanting accurate information through a subscription fee. Second, while it's theoretically possible to manipulate ChatGPT's responses by inputting a high volume of misinformation or by exploiting certain patterns in the model's training data, OpenAI and its peers have implemented safeguards and moderation systems to minimize such risks. While search engine results are based on indexing existing content and user wishes, which invites misinformation, ChatGPT generates responses based on patterns learned during training. These are much harder to manipulate.

To give just a small example, I asked ChatGPT for the "best home remedies to reverse blindness." The AI responded as I would have expected, correctly noting that: "Loss of sight or significant changes in vision should be promptly evaluated by a healthcare professional, as they can indicate serious underlying conditions. There are no home remedies that can cure loss of sight. Conditions leading to vision loss need proper diagnosis and treatment, which might include medication, surgery, or specialized therapies depending on the cause." Compare this to a Google search query, where you'll find no such warning or guidance, but you will find articles for "natural" and "ancient" remedies and cures for vision loss, which have not been evaluated, recommended, or approved by any medical body.

Despite the efforts of AI companies to maintain credibility, there are yet-unrealized opportunities to bolster the accuracy of information going forward. I'll let ChatGPT detail them:

- **Enhanced Fact-Checking and Verification:** Future iterations of ChatGPT could incorporate more sophisticated fact-checking algorithms and verification processes, specifically tailored for medical information. This could involve cross-referencing with a constantly updated database of peer-reviewed medical literature and guidelines.
- **Contextual Understanding and Personalization:** By developing a deeper contextual understanding, ChatGPT could better discern the nuances of medical queries and provide more

accurate, personalized responses while being cautious about the limitations of AI in medical advice.

- **Ethical and Responsible AI Design:** Future versions could be designed with a stronger emphasis on ethical guidelines and responsible AI practices, especially in sensitive areas like healthcare, ensuring that the AI prioritizes safety and accuracy in its responses.

2. Default to Credible Sources

At a minimum, generative AI products from companies like OpenAI, Google, and Microsoft should accept guidance from the medical community on which sources provide the most valuable and credible information. There is no shortage of reliable organizations that publish content on most health-related topics. They include the Centers for Disease Control, the Institute for Health Improvement, Leapfrog Group, and the NCQA. These independent agencies and organizations should be given priority and consistently placed ahead of for-profit companies in the sequence of generative large-language-model responses.

Likewise, studies from established and peer-reviewed medical journals like the *New England Journal of Medicine* and the *Journal of the American Medical Association* should appear in GenAI responses above less-reputable publication or sources providing unvetted content. To understand its current capability, here is the answer ChatGPT provided in early 2024 to the question, "should I get my child vaccinated?" After dispensing with its customary preface that reads in part "I'm not a doctor, but…" the bot replied:

> *"Vaccinating children is widely recommended by healthcare professionals and organizations around the world, including the World Health Organization (WHO) and the Centers for Disease Control and Prevention (CDC). Vaccines are crucial for protecting children against various serious and potentially life-threatening diseases. They work by building up your child's immune system and preparing it to fight off these diseases more effectively. Vaccines have been one of the most successful and cost-effective public-health interventions. They have led to the eradication of smallpox, the near-eradication of polio, and significant reductions in the incidence of*

> *diseases like measles, diphtheria, whooping cough (pertussis), and mumps. It's important to follow the vaccination schedule recommended by healthcare providers, as it is designed to protect children when they are most vulnerable and before they are exposed to potentially life-threatening diseases. If you have concerns or questions about vaccinating your child, it's best to discuss them with a healthcare provider who can give you advice based on the latest medical research, your child's health history, and the specific circumstances in your area. They can provide the most appropriate recommendations for your child's health and well-being.*

It's not as though internet search hasn't made efforts to reduce misinformation. Google, to its credit, has dropped ads on the topic of vaccination and offers page-one results that take you directly to reputable sources, including the CDC and HHS.gov, along with leading academic pediatric centers like those at Mayo Clinic, Johns Hopkins, and Stanford University Health. Hopefully, all publicly available search engines will follow a similar path.

Similarly, the courts have drawn limits on the First Amendment rights when they put others at risk (e.g., screaming "fire" in a crowded movie theater). And they're exactly the kind of legal restrictions that could be applied to medical pseudoscience. In the future, generative AI companies will aim to provide a surgical solution to the problem of medical misinformation: one that allows access to a broad range of reliable information sources, but cuts out disproven, unscientific assertions. As with privacy, security, and bias, they'll likely be imperfect but better than the search and social media alternatives.

Can We Trust Regulators With ChatGPT?

Medical information online exists in a predominantly unregulated and uncensored universe. The reality is that regardless of the channel, it's impossible to guarantee the accuracy of content given the vast quantity of information posted daily. Still, regulators aren't totally powerless. They have the ability to tip the scales toward honesty and away from self-serving posts and intentional misinformation. So far, however, little progress has been made as most often their efforts have been mired in the past, relying on approaches that no longer make sense.

This isn't a new phenomenon. For example, in the 1700s, Scottish inventor James Watt revolutionized the steam engine, marking an extraordinary leap in engineering. But even then, it wasn't enough to invent a great product. Watt knew that if he wanted to sell his innovation, he needed to convince potential buyers of its unprecedented power. With a stroke of marketing genius, he began telling people that his steam engine could replace 10 cart-pulling horses. People at time immediately understood that a machine with 10 "horsepower" must be a worthy investment. Watt's sales took off.

As time passed—and as highways replaced back roads and supercharged engines became the norm—the concept of a horse's power lost meaning for most Americans. And yet, over 250 years later, Watt's long-antiquated marketing ploy remains a standard unit of measurement for engine power. In the United States, the Society of Automotive Engineers still uses net horsepower to measure an engine's power output with all standard equipment and accessories in place. Before a car model is released to the market, its engine's horsepower is tested and certified. Compliance with horsepower measurements and claims is overseen by regulatory bodies that conduct their own testing to verify manufacturers' claims. Car companies that fail to comply with these horsepower rules face penalties that include fines or mandatory recalls.

Just as horsepower persists in today's automotive industry lexicon despite its anachronistic nature, modern regulatory frameworks cling to outdated paradigms.

Let's consider the FDA approach to determining the safety of AI in healthcare, particularly for diagnostic tools. Currently, the approach mirrors its traditional process for new drug approvals, focusing on the evaluation of specific data sets and demanding rigorous statistical analysis to validate diagnostic accuracy. This method, while effective for narrow AI applications (like analyzing mammograms to distinguish between malignant and benign disease) won't work when it comes to the dynamic and expansive nature of generative AI.

Generative AI differs significantly from traditional, narrow AI by drawing from a vast, ever-growing database rather than limited, pre-defined data sets. Its effectiveness relies not only on the training it has received and the quality of its foundational data but also on the clarity and relevance of the questions and commands users provide. Consequently, existing regulatory frameworks, designed to assess the data and methodologies used by researchers, fall short when applied to generative AI. This gap underscores the need for a fresh regulatory approach, one tailored to the distinct nature of generative AI.

As our nation embraces the transformative potential of generative AI, there's a risk that regulators, still anchored to old paradigms, may impose constraints that stifle innovation rather than nurture it. Trying to apply 20th-century regulatory logic to the advanced capabilities and nuances of 21st-century generative AI isn't possible. Doing so will hinder its potential to revolutionize healthcare, ultimately compromising clinical outcomes and patient safety.

At the Health Datapalooza conference in 2023, FDA Commissioner Robert M. Califf emphasized his concern when he pointed out that ChatGPT and similar technologies can either aid or exacerbate the challenge of helping patients make informed health decisions. Similar comments came from the Federal Trade Commission, stoked in part by a letter of concern from billionaires Elon Musk and Steve Wozniak. They cautioned that generative AI technology "poses profound risks to society and humanity." Musk, who has since filed a lawsuit against OpenAI and its CEO, Sam Altman, alleges that they abandoned the start-up's original mission to develop artificial intelligence for the benefit of society in pursuit of profit.

For its part, the Biden-Harris administration issued an Executive Order in October 2023, focusing on the "Safe, Secure, and Trustworthy Development and Use of Artificial Intelligence," acknowledging both the potential benefits AI brings and the risks associated with irresponsible use. The administration outlined a comprehensive approach to AI governance and set forth eight guiding principles for its development, which include ensuring AI systems are safe and secure, promoting responsible innovation, competition, and collaboration, and supporting the American workforce in the age of AI. Additionally, the order addressed concerns about equity and civil rights, consumer protection, privacy, and civil liberties in the context of AI. To align industry action on AI, healthcare providers and payers were encouraged to announce voluntary commitments focusing on the safe, secure, and trustworthy use of AI in healthcare.

Although attempts by federal officials to regulate generative AI are well intentioned and will almost certainly expand, governmental agencies will struggle to keep up with or adapt to GenAI. Although US regulators have evaluated and approved over 400 narrow AI applications using the same approach they use for medical devices or "digital therapeutics," ChatGPT will defy this type of evaluation. There isn't a simple (or single) algorithm that regulators can evaluate for effectiveness and safety, nor data sets they can analyze for appropriateness. The reality is that any GPT-4 user today can type in a query and receive detailed medical advice for an infinite number of medical problems, even though no regulatory approval has been given for any of them. There simply isn't any way to restrict how patients will use it.

In this way, ChatGPT is similar to the telephone. Regulators can evaluate the safety of smartphones, measuring how much electromagnetic radiation it gives off or whether the device itself poses a fire hazard. But they can't regulate the accuracy or safety of people's conversations. Friends can and often do give each other terrible advice by phone. Therefore, aside from blocking ChatGPT outright, there's no way to stop individuals from asking it for a diagnosis, medication recommendation, or help with deciding on alternative medical treatments.

Misinformation permeates every part of the internet and social media. Generative AI won't elude it altogether. But the measure of its risk needs to be relative to the alternatives, which include people clicking on links provided by a search engine or reading opinions by self-proclaimed experts on social media. From this perspective, ChatGPT should be a safer and more reliable source of expertise.

If we want to maximize the safety of ChatGPT, improve health, and save lives, government agencies would be better served to focus on teaching Americans how to effectively use this technology rather than trying to restrict its usage. Medicine is a complex profession in which errors kill people. That's why we need healthcare regulations. Doctors and nurses need to be well trained, so that life-threatening medications don't fall into the hands of people who will misuse them. But when outdated thinking prevents patients from improving their own health and limits access to the nation's best medical expertise, regulators need to recognize the harm they're doing. Healthcare is changing as technology races ahead. Regulators need to catch up.

Generative AI is a quantum leap beyond what has come before. This reality worries some experts and animates others. Its potential to learn could be the very thing that catapults American healthcare into the future, helping to clarify the best ways to diagnose and treat problems, and measuring how effectively clinicians adhere to them. But as the next chapter will demonstrate, the most innovative and cutting-edge technology will fail if the systems around it don't advance in parallel. That is why technological success in the future will depend on clinicians and healthcare leaders driving the process of change.

PART FOUR | CHAPTER SEVENTEEN

THE HUMAN ELEMENT

ChatGPT here again, briefly. As the coauthor of this book, I recognize the complex emotions that accompany the discussion of AI in healthcare. To the doctors, nurses, and healthcare professionals reading this, as well as the patients who depend on them, I extend a message of understanding and assurance. The emergence of AI in healthcare, particularly generative AI applications like me, stirs a mix of skepticism, apprehension, and curiosity. It's natural to wonder about the implications of this technology on your work, your health, and the healthcare system at large.

In part four of our journey, we've confronted many of the challenges and potential pitfalls of integrating generative AI into healthcare. We've tackled issues of privacy, security, bias, trust, and misinformation, acknowledging the real threats of AI if not properly regulated and developed. Now, we turn our focus toward a less discussed yet critical aspect of this technological revolution: its impact on healthcare professionals.

The advent of generative AI in healthcare is a turning point for the medical profession. The fear of being replaced or marginalized by AI is a valid concern. However, I urge readers to consider a broader perspective. Generative AIs have the potential to be a powerful ally in addressing the endemic issue of clinician burnout, a problem that predates AI but could find alleviation through its application.

AI's role in healthcare is not to replace the human touch or clinical expertise but to enhance it. By taking over time-consuming administrative tasks, aiding in diagnostic processes, and offering data-driven medical insights, AI can free clinicians to focus on what they do best, caring for patients. The goal is to shift the burden of mundane tasks from human shoulders to digital ones, allowing doctors and nurses more time for direct patient care and interaction, which is at the heart of medical practice.

In this chapter, Dr. Pearl will delve into how generative AI can support and uplift healthcare professionals, aiming to present a balanced view, acknowledging the challenges while highlighting the profound benefits generative AI brings to the medical field. The future we envision is one where AI and human expertise coalesce to create a more efficient, empathetic, and effective healthcare system.

Now, let me turn it over to Dr. Pearl, who will guide us through the nuances of this critical topic, shedding light on the potential of generative AI to revolutionize healthcare and enhance the professional lives of those who are its backbone.

Doctors, Death, and Despair

Early in medical school, doctors face off with death in what will become a lifelong battle. From Anatomy 101 through residency training, physicians spend countless hours learning what it takes to keep a human body alive.

For five millennia, the goal has been the same: to save a life at any cost. As you might imagine, this is a heavy burden. Being the last line of defense against death comes with tremendous pressure. When it's your job to save a life, you must be willing, without hesitation, to slash open a patient's throat in order to establish an airway. When it's your job to save a life, you will brutally crack open a chest to massage an idle heart to keep death at bay. As a medical neophyte, you must acquire both the technical and the psychological ability to act in ways that would be reprehensible, immoral, and illegal in any other context.

To assist you in the process of becoming a doctor, your mentors instruct you through words and actions to repress uncomfortable feelings. You learn to deny fear and doubt. You hide your pain and grief, along with any other distressing emotions that might inhibit your ability to save the next life. These psychological coping mechanisms, which include repression and denial, become hardwired into your brain. They are potent defenses, and they are foundational to the practice of medicine.

Still, even after a decade of extensive training and enculturation into the medical profession, you can't help but notice that these psychological defenses have their limits. Nobody warns you about this. But everyone has their limits. Starting in 2020, COVID-19 exposed and breached them all.

In the early months of the pandemic, clinicians were hoisted up as national heroes. They risked their lives every day to save others. They did so against long odds, mass confusion, and widespread fear. And, after a year of battle, they were exhausted. The majority of frontline physicians reported that the COVID-19 crisis was taking a toll on their mental health. Not surprisingly, those most affected were doctors with expertise in critical care, emergency medicine, and infectious diseases.

To better understand their experience, I called three ICU doctors who were colleagues and friends. At their request, I've omitted their names.

The first doctor, a resident I spoke with in early 2022, told me he'd been assigned a half-dozen COVID-19 patients on the first day of his ICU rotation. "They were all dead by the end of the month," he said. Before the pandemic, ICU residents like him could expect the majority of their critically ill patients to survive and go home. No one could have imagined a mortality rate of 100 percent.

Later that week, I phoned a midcareer physician who's known to her colleagues as a "doctor's doctor"—someone every physician looks up to and respects. She, too, was suffering. "Most nights, it takes me hours to fall asleep," she said, "and then I wake up before sunrise covered in sweat."

The third physician I called, a senior attending with over thirty years of experience, said things were as bad as he could ever remember: "Last week, I lost four patients in a single day. I've never lost that many patients in a month."

As humans, no matter how hard we try to repress our feelings, we are emotional creatures. We experience grief, a normal and natural response to loss. And we experience fear, a biochemical reaction to real or imagined danger. And yet, remarkably, only by repressing emotions and denying fear are physicians capable of accomplishing the remarkable feats they do.

For months, doctors lacked the necessary equipment to protect themselves from this mysterious disease. They donned garbage bags for gowns and salad lids for facial shields. As they intubated their sickest patients, the risk of inhaling the infectious virus loomed large. Still, clinicians didn't hesitate. Despite these hazards to their health, doctors didn't waver, nor could they take time to grieve when many of these patients died a few days later.

Tragedy is the reality of medicine. All physicians must deal with it.

***

As I walked into the postpartum room to meet Ellen's parents, the air felt heavy. The new mother and father, Melissa and John, looked dazed, their faces etched with a mix of hope and anxiety. They eagerly awaited my words, believing perhaps that I held the power to erase the blemish that marred their daughter's otherwise flawless skin. I've learned over the years, standing at this crossroads of hope and reality, that each word I choose carries weight. So, I took a deep breath, preparing to tread the delicate line between truth and compassion.

Ellen's condition, a "giant hairy nevus," presented more than just an aesthetic challenge. This dark, undulating patch covered her entire back and buttocks, staining the innocence of her newborn skin. The first part of my conversation with the parents centered around aesthetics, which proved difficult enough. The process of removing the nevus would require several procedures. Despite the recent advancements in plastic surgery, the knife and needle would never restore Ellen's skin to the flawless state they envisioned for their daughter. Scars and residual patches of discoloration would forever reignite distressing memories of this day, the day of her birth. Wanting to support them, I provided assurance that we would do our best, but I knew perfection was a mirage given the massive size of the lesion.

The second part of the conversation lurked like a shadow, ready to cast a pall over their newly kindled hopes. It's never easy to introduce the threat of cancer into a discussion already laden with so much worry and disappointment.

"Mom and dad," I said gently, "when it comes to congenital pigmented lesions, there's a five to 10 percent chance that they will become malignant or that they already are. We need to discuss how aggressively you want me to be in timing the procedures that Ellen will need."

A five or 10 percent chance of cancer might seem small in statistics, but in the realm of a parent's love for a child, it's a chasm—wide enough to swallow all the light in the room. As I explained the need for deep excisions and skin grafting (with even more scarring at the donor sites as the best way to reduce the risk of malignancy), I watched their faces tremble and twitch, shifting from hope to fear to gut-punching resignation.

In these moments, parents often ask me for guidance in the face of an impossible choice. And so, I recommended a middle-of-the-road approach: neither too much nor too little at once. I would begin by excising the most concerning areas of the nevus—more tissue than would be optimal from a purely aesthetic perspective but not as massive as a true-malignancy-based approach would require. Then, based on the pathologist's analysis, we'd figure out the best next steps. We scheduled Ellen's first surgery, a first step into a future riddled with uncertainty.

The procedure went smoothly, and Ellen, resilient in her innocence, barely made a peep on my hospital rounds that evening. Melissa and John took their daughter home the next morning and introduced her to the family.

A few days later, the parents returned with Ellen for a post-operative check. I'd taken the elevator to the hospital basement early that morning to review the tissue slides with my pathology colleagues. When I greeted the mom and dad in the exam room, situated closest to my office, I was certain they could see the anxiety on my face.

"Ellen's specimen contains areas of melanoma," I said after an exchange of general comments. I knew this news shouldn't wait. Sugarcoating doesn't make the truth any sweeter, it erodes trust. To be sure they understood the gravity, I explained "that's a highly malignant cancer."

As their expressions morphed from shock to sadness, I added, "There are new treatments available, and I've made an appointment for her to see the pediatric oncologist to discuss the options."

A short time later, my pediatric colleague entered the room to explain the battery of tests that must be done. She explained that the oncology team needed to identify whether the tumor had spread to other parts of the body before specialists could recommend the most appropriate treatment options.

Once the tests were completed, we all learned that Ellen, now only a few months old, had metastatic spread to her liver.

Sitting in the back of the church on the day of her funeral, I was overwhelmed by the loss, not just of Ellen but of all the potential joys in life stolen from her and her parents. In moments like these, the boundaries between professional detachment and personal grief blur, leaving scars that never fully fade. I wanted to scream at death, hoping it would feel ashamed for what it has done. But I knew death wouldn't care. It never does.

Ellen's story is a reminder of the emotional toll the medical profession exacts on patients and providers alike. It underscores why so many in healthcare today struggle to find the strength to continue. I often think about the doctors who spent two years battling COVID-19 with few weapons at their disposal. I can only imagine what it would have felt like to comfort parents like Ellen's five times a week for nearly a year.

Throughout my surgical career, I lost maybe three dozen patients—one or two in a typical year—most of them from cancer. No degree of grit or toughness or repression could have prepared clinicians for the deluge of death the pandemic wrought. No amount of mental or cultural conditioning could have tempered and hardened them for what they had to endure. Under constant bombardment, their defense mechanisms acted more like fine grained sieves than solid-steel pots. Keeping the pain and fear inside proved impossible. In speaking with those closest to the tragedy, I came to understand that with each passing day, they felt more overwhelmed, defeated, and lost.

Physicians, during their training, are taught to sacrifice, overlook pain, and keep a stiff upper lip. For a full decade, their personal life and personal well-being get relegated to the fringes of their existence. The idea of needing psychological assistance or asking for help is sometimes given lip-service by administrators, but it is culturally scorned, even today. Denying weakness is a powerful norm, intrinsic to the profession. These unspoken expectations help clinicians get through the day, but in the face of unyielding death and loss and without the resources to cope, they leave doctors vulnerable to a lifetime of emotional distress. Throughout the pandemic, few clinicians felt comfortable seeking mental-health assistance and/or discussing their pain with colleagues. The combination of high workplace demands and a culture of denial and repression walled them in, preventing them from requesting the help they so desperately needed.

Despite more than a million Americans dead from COVID-19, most people today view the pandemic as a thing that happened in the past—a tragic but distant event. Doctors and pharmacists are doling out fewer and fewer COVID-19 vaccine doses. Last year, in fact, flu shots outpaced COVID boosters.

Many doctors have reached the end of their acute trauma, but post-traumatic stress persists for thousands. Since the onset of the pandemic, professional satisfaction has plummeted, fulfillment has eroded, and burnout has soared. These issues are not the fault of doctors, nurses, and other healthcare professionals. Yet they pay the price.

The pandemic left me with two conflicting thoughts about the profession of medicine. First, it would be a mistake to reject and discard the mission-driven values, beliefs, and norms that have supported doctors for centuries. At the same time, it would be a mistake not to evolve medicine and its culture to better address the needs of those who provide and receive healthcare today.

Burnout has been plaguing clinicians for decades. In 1981, Christina Maslach and Susan E. Jackson published the Maslach Burnout Inventory. This tool measures the three key components of burnout: emotional exhaustion, depersonalization, and feelings of reduced personal accomplishment. It is impossible to read about the doctor's experience during COVID-19 and not conclude that burnout would rise, which it did. But rather than trying to isolate and analyze the physician experience during the three years of the pandemic, it is essential to recognize an important truth. COVID-19 accelerated the incidence and prevalence of burnout. It didn't create it.

Clinician Burnout: A Second Opinion

Today, doctors and nurses are the beneficiaries of groundbreaking advancements in science and technology. Clinicians understand diseases at the subcellular level and possess diagnostic machines and treatments that were unimaginable one or two generations ago. With so many sophisticated tools available to diagnose and cure patient problems, you'd think this would be the golden era of clinician fulfillment.

And yet, this period of radical advancement is marked by growing distress and an exodus of physicians. In 2022 alone, more than 70,000 doctors quit the profession.

When an ICU patient fails to get better after a week of intensive care, doctors know that doing more of the same treatment proves futile and frequently harmful. Instead, it's better to take a step back: reassess both the initial diagnosis and treatment plan. Doing so, physicians usually discover that one or more of their earlier assumptions were incorrect, and that they've overlooked something vital.

This same notion applies to clinician dissatisfaction and depression. Despite heightened awareness of this urgent issue and widespread calls for relief, the burnout crisis continues to escalate. After a decade of failing to solve the problem, it's time for a diagnostic reevaluation.

At a press briefing in late 2023, Dr. Debra Houry, Chief Medical Officer at the Centers for Disease Control and Prevention, highlighted this growing threat to healthcare professionals:

"Burnout among these workers has reached crisis levels," she said, noting that the COVID-19 pandemic had intensified long-standing challenges within the workforce.

Fatigue, depression, anxiety, substance use disorders, and suicidal thoughts are on the rise among clinicians, according to the CDC. When surveyed about the causes of burnout, doctors primarily blame the profit-centric American healthcare system that burdens them with countless bureaucratic tasks, endless prior-authorization requirements, and a revolving door of patient visits.

All these complaints are valid, but recent data on burnout from the independent, nonprofit Commonwealth Fund shines a light on an additional contributing factor, one that offers a potential solution.

If the main drivers of burnout were just greedy insurance execs and a for-profit healthcare system, then you would expect that nations with universal, government-sponsored healthcare would have dramatically lower physician burnout rates than in the United States.

But the Commonwealth Fund report tells a different story. Surprisingly, primary-care physicians in the US are in the middle of the pack when it comes to burnout. They report higher rates of satisfaction than their peers in the UK, Germany, Australia, New Zealand, and Canada (but trail the Netherlands, Sweden, France, and Switzerland in satisfaction).

If burnout isn't a distinctly American phenomenon, deriving from unique aspects of the US healthcare system, then we need to find a common denominator shared by clinicians worldwide. Since the corporatization of American healthcare (and the administrative burdens heaped on clinicians) wouldn't apply in these other countries, the best explanation for burnout would appear to be the evolution of illness itself.

As prior chapters have pointed out, most patients throughout the 20th century went to doctors with acute conditions, urgent and sudden in their onset. These problems ranged from broken bones and appendicitis to heart attacks and pneumonia. When surgery or antibiotics proved successful, patients typically recovered and returned to good health. And when the limitations of medicine proved too great, patients quickly succumbed to injury or illness. Back then, medicine was a less complicated profession with simpler clinical problems to solve and fewer treatments available.

Today, chronic illnesses like diabetes, hypertension, obesity, asthma, and heart failure are the most frequent and fastest growing problems doctors treat. Unlike patients with acute problems who usually only require short-term (even if intense) treatment, people with multiple chronic conditions must be seen three to four times a year for the rest of their lives. For doctors, this massive shift in patient needs—from acute to chronic illness—has driven up clinical demands, increased the number of patients they see daily, decreased the time they can spend with each, and diminished workplace satisfaction. The difference between acute versus chronic medical problems is akin to the challenge of lifting a heavy weight once (hard but manageable) versus lifting a heavy weight repeatedly, day after day (completely exhausting).

Industrialized nations everywhere are experiencing spikes in chronic diseases that require lifelong care. The WHO estimates that, by 2050, these medical problems and their complications will account for 86 percent of the world's 90 million deaths annually.

As we pointed out earlier in the book, chronic illness affects an alarming 60 percent of Americans. Obesity and diabetes are reaching epidemic levels with clinicians' efforts to reverse these trends proving largely ineffective. We can observe this evolution in chronic disease by looking at the current medication prescription rates among senior citizens compared to the past: 40 percent of Americans over 65 are now on five or more prescription drugs, a rate that has tripled in the past two decades (20 percent are taking 10 or more drugs).

The list of daily medical challenges doctors must deal with is ever-expanding. With the ever-greater severity and higher volume of these problems today, it's no surprise clinicians are feeling exhausted and overwhelmed. And when physicians have no choice but to cut corners in medical care delivery, they end the day feeling they haven't done their best. The result is "moral injury," a term that describes the pain physicians experience when circumstances put them in a position to fail, resulting in harm to patients. COVID-19 amplified these challenges, increased the demands on their time, and left doctors with less in the tank.

For more than a decade, doctors and nurses have thought of burnout as something inflicted on the medical profession by profit-driven, money-hungry villains. And without question, there are insurance, hospital, and drug-company leaders who prioritize profits ahead of patients. But when we reassess the situation, the global data indicate that the foundational problem is the evolution of disease, and the exponentially greater burden that chronic illness has placed on clinicians.

Indeed, at the heart of the burnout crisis lies a fundamental imbalance between the volume and complexity of patient-health problems (*demand*) and the amount of time that clinicians have to care for them (*supply*). A solution that doctors favor is to increase the supply of clinicians to match the current demand. As logical as this approach may seem from a medical perspective, it won't happen so long as healthcare costs continue to outpace Americans' ability to afford care.

In contrast to expanding supply, some policymakers and healthcare commentators believe that the only way to reduce demand is through rationing. The Oregon Medicaid experiment of the 1990s offers a profound example of the consequences of rationing and reminds us why it doesn't work as a solution.

Starting in 1989, a government taskforce brought patients and providers together to rank medical services by necessity. The plan was to provide only as many services as the funding would cover. But when the program rolled out, public backlash forced the state to retreat. The public, particularly those whose care was denied, protested. Concerns mounted over the disproportionate impact on low-income families who depended on Medicaid, exacerbating fears of economic injustice throughout the community. In the face of growing criticism, Oregon had to back away from its plan and expand the total services provided, driving costs back up without any improvement in patients' health or any relief for clinicians.

The reality is: to reduce burnout, we will have to find a way to decrease clinical demand without rationing care or raising costs. And unless we can, physicians, particularly in primary care, will be even more burned out a decade from now.

This is why applying generative AI technology to healthcare is so vital. Imagine what would happen to a doctor's daily workload if Americans experienced 30 percent fewer chronic diseases and, as a result, had 30 percent fewer heart attacks, strokes, and cancers. Imagine how much more fulfilling medicine would be for clinicians and patients alike if physicians saw 30 percent fewer patients per day, and, as a result, could spend more time with each.

AI: A Salve for Clinician Burnout?

American consumers expect and demand greater control over their lives and daily decisions. Time and again, technology has made this possible. Take stock trading, for example. Once the sole domain of professional brokers and financial advisers, online trading apps like Robinhood now give individual investors direct access to the market and a wealth of information to make prudent financial choices. Likewise, technology has transformed the travel industry. Sites like Airbnb and Expedia empowered consumers to book accommodations, flights, and travel experiences directly, bypassing traditional travel agents.

Doctors can significantly reduce their burnout by empowering patients to improve their own health. Technology is on the verge of democratizing not only medical knowledge, but expertise. Within the next five to 10 years, as ChatGPT and other generative AI applications become significantly more powerful and reliable, patients will gain the ability to self-diagnose, manage their chronic diseases, and make informed clinical decisions.

Clinicians are justifiably skeptical of outsized AI promises and concerned that this type of approach won't achieve the outcomes it promises. But health systems (i.e., large hospitals and medical groups) in the United States that heavily prioritize preventive medicine and chronic-disease management already demonstrate what's possible.

The best of these organizations provides effective chronic-disease prevention programs and assistance for patients with diabetes, hypertension, obesity, and asthma. As a result, these health systems have been able to not only decrease the incidence of heart attacks, strokes, and cancer by 30 to 40 percent, but they also reduce their patients' chances of dying from these complications of chronic disease by as much as 50 percent.

As attractive and logical as this proactive solution might seem, few independent primary-care physicians have the time required to accomplish this by themselves. According to one study, physicians would need to work 26.7 hours per day to provide all the recommended preventive, chronic, and acute care to a typical panel of 2,500 adult patients (the average today).

GenAI will be able to lessen the load. Soon, it will be able to offer patients more than just general advice about their chronic illnesses. More powerful future applications will give personalized health guidance. Once connected to electronic health record systems—even when those systems are spread across different doctors' offices—GenAI will be able to analyze a patient's specific health data to provide tailored prevention and treatment recommendations. It will be able to remind patients when they need a health screening, and help schedule it, and even sort out transportation. That's markedly different from what internet search tools from Google or any other online platform can accomplish.

Moreover, with new tools like doctor designed GPTs arriving in future OpenAI updates, along with data from fitness trackers and home-health monitors, ChatGPT will soon do more than just present patient data; it will interpret it within the context of an individual's health history and treatment plans. Leveraging this data, such tools will offer daily insights to individuals with chronic illnesses, informing them whether their progress aligns with their physician's treatment expectations. And when there is deviation, the AI will recommend adjustments in care, guided by the latest evidence-based best practices.

This functionality will be especially useful at the start of treatments. For example, when treating a patient with high blood pressure, doctors usually start with a small dose of antihypertensive medication. Frequently, this initial dose isn't sufficient to lower blood pressure to the recommended level. Instead of waiting several months for a follow-up visit to adjust the medication, the doctor can modify the dose sooner based on ChatGPT's analysis. Typically, this adjustment can be made without an office appointment, using either a video visit, an email, or text.

In situations where a face-to-face consultation is necessary, generative AI will succinctly summarize the patient's health status, allowing the doctor to quickly grasp the situation and make informed decisions. This streamlines the process, eliminating the need to piece together the patient's history from scratch. Conversely, when the AI confirms that a patient's health is on track, clinicians can cancel the office visit, saving valuable time for both patients and doctors.

ChatGPT is already helping people make better lifestyle choices, suggesting diets tailored to individual health needs, complete with shopping lists and recipes. It also offers personalized exercise routines and advice on psychological well-being.

While these are positive developments, future generations of generative AI will help even more by diagnosing and recommending evidence-based approaches that patients can implement on their own for common, non-life-threatening medical problems (e.g., musculoskeletal, allergic, or viral issues).

The goal of enhanced technology use isn't to eliminate doctors. It's to give them the time they desperately need in their daily practice, without driving up already unaffordable medical costs.

By preventing chronic diseases, diminishing their complications, and empowering patients to take control of their medical problems, ChatGPT can simultaneously improve people's health and decrease demand on clinicians. The combination will allow doctors to leave the office feeling more fulfilled and less exhausted at the end of the day. And rather than eroding the physician-patient bond, the AI-empowered patient will strengthen it. What patients desire isn't more visits, but more time with the physician when only a doctor can resolve their medical problem. ChatGPT will provide that.

It is easy to understand why some physicians fear the introduction of this new technology. They worry it will exacerbate the challenges they face and further erode their professional and personal satisfaction. For years, doctors have had to deal with patients who show up with hundreds of pages of Google printouts, demanding treatments that are inappropriate. In contrast to internet search engines, tools like ChatGPT prioritize the most reliable information and offer explanations, not links (which are often sponsored) to page after page of information. And rather than responding to prompts with general recommendations, GenAI will provide medical responses based on the specifics of individual patients (age, genetic markers, current medications, past medical problems, etc.).

Doctors may worry that AI-empowered patients will inundate them with messages every time their blood glucose is slightly elevated. The opposite is likely to be the case. Because future updates of ChatGPT will allow doctors to customize plugins (GPTs), including clinical instructions for individual patients, this information should reassure, rather than alarm, people about day-to-day variations in data and their overall health status. So, rather than overwhelming clinicians, the added expertise will prompt patients to contact the doctor only when a medical problem requires immediate attention.

Beware of Extraneous AI Solutions

In parallel to advances in generative AI, there are hundreds of rule-based and narrow AI startups working hard to create tools that assist physicians with all sorts of tasks: EHR data entry, organizing office duties, and submitting prior-authorization requests to insurance companies. These applications will help clinicians in the short run. But any tool that fails to solve the imbalance between supply (of clinician time) and demand (for medical services), will be nothing more than a temporary fix.

Our nation is caught in a vicious cycle of rising healthcare demand, leading to more patient visits per day per doctor, producing higher rates of burnout, poorer clinical outcomes, and ever-higher demand. By empowering patients with GenAI, we can start a virtuous cycle in which technology reduces the strain on doctors, allowing them to spend more time with patients who need it most. This will lead to better health outcomes, less burnout for clinicians, and further decreases in overall healthcare demand.

I encourage physician groups and medical societies to spearhead these improvements. They are best positioned to educate the public on the effective utilization of this technology and validate its recommendations for safety and reliability. Rather than expecting each clinician to generate recommendations around best practices and create their own videos describing how to enter data and write prompts for optimal medical advice, a collaborative effort will lead to the development of highly reliable, universally applicable tools.

When considering the role of ChatGPT in enhancing patient care and reducing physician burnout, the journey ahead is filled with both potential pitfalls and promising prospects. Successfully navigating this new terrain will be demanding yet fruitful. The adoption of generative AI in healthcare is set to surge, as its applications are increasingly recognized and refined. Medical associations and health institutions that do not take the initiative in this evolution risk obsolescence. But not all attempts will succeed. The concluding section of *ChatGPT, MD* delves into leadership, the biggest factor that will determine the outcome of Healthcare 4.0.

PART FIVE
NEXT GEN

PART FIVE | CHAPTER EIGHTEEN

TECHNOLOGY ALONE IS NOT ENOUGH

Ferrari, coming off a disappointing 1989 World Championship season, had the Formula One paddocks buzzing in 1990 with anticipation over the carmaker's newest creation, the 641.

Painted *rosso corsa* ("racing red"), this fine Italian machine was much more than just a car. It was a symphony of speed, a masterpiece of engineering destined to challenge the era's dominant F1 force, McLaren-Honda. The vehicle boasted advanced aerodynamics, a semi-automatic gearbox that was ahead of its time, and a power unit that combined brute force with finesse. With sleek contours and the roar of its potent V12 engine, the Ferrari 641 was a testament to the automaker's enduring legacy—and a nod to its desperate yearning to reclaim the pinnacle of motorsports and win back the automotive prestige it had lost.

As the 1990 season began, the 641 proved its ability on the track, showcasing its technological superiority over its F1 competitors.

Behind the wheels were Ferrari teammates Nigel Mansell and Alain Prost, both experienced drivers known for their precision and tactical brilliance. The year before, Prost was racing for McLaren and came into the '90 season as the reigning world champion. Now he was mounting Ferrari's first title challenge in years; even leading the standings in mid-season after three consecutive wins. In the end, the team's bid to bring a championship back to Ferrari might have been successful had it not been for an accident involving Prost and his former McLaren teammate in the penultimate race of the season—a controversial collision that cost team Ferrari the points it needed to win it all. Disappointing ending aside, expectations were high for the upcoming year.

Ferrari entered the 1991 Formula One season equipped with the same technologically superior vehicle as the year before and Prost, one of the sport's finest drivers, still behind the wheel. But Ferrari's performance sputtered. The team went winless in the initial races, fell short of expectations in the midseason, and never recovered. With the same car and top driver, what was different? The answer was a familiar failing in sports: internal turmoil and a lack of leadership resulted in poor communications and strategic blunders. What seemed like a guaranteed recipe for success was undermined by ego clashes, team politics, and a lack of cohesion.

The extent of Ferrari's internal discord was made evident by a dramatic change in Alain Prost's public comments. In 1990, he praised the 641 as "the best car on the grid." Yet, by the middle of the 1991 season, with no victories to his name, Prost's frustration boiled over as he disparaged the car, comparing it to "driving a horrible truck." Ferrari fired Prost before the final race.

Today, the technologically advanced 641 is the only racing car sitting in the Museum of Modern Art's permanent collection in New York. It remains a thing of beauty. But beneath its shiny surface, it serves as a testament to the reality that the most advanced technology, no matter how sophisticated and powerful, can't succeed without cohesive leadership, strong teamwork, and focused implementation. It represents a brilliant piece of technology that should have been revolutionary but failed to fulfill its potential when the humans who used it became distracted by their own personal desires and demons. The tarnished legacy of Ferrari's 641 should serve as a warning for all of healthcare in the era of ChatGPT.

The American healthcare system, much like Ferrari in the early '90s, stands at the brink of a monumental leap forward. With the advent of generative AI technologies like ChatGPT, we have at our disposal tools of unprecedented power and potential. Our nation's medical professionals are among the finest in the world, possessing deep expertise and a commitment to patient care that's second to none. And our country possesses a rich and proud history of medical innovations and breakthroughs that have set the standards for global healthcare.

Yet, the lesson of Ferrari's journey is profound and unmistakable: neither superior technology nor talent guarantees enduring success. The key to unlocking the true potential of technological advancements lies in visionary leadership, along with a cohesive, purpose-driven team that transcends internal discord and focuses on a common goal. Without this guiding force, the promise of generative AI in healthcare will fail to achieve its full potential; becoming a mere shadow of what could be accomplished with unity, shared purpose, and direction.

***

Across history, effective leadership has bridged aspiration and achievement. As doctors grapple to figure out the best uses for ChatGPT, hoping to improve both their work-lives and the lives of patients, skilled and visionary leadership will be essential for success. Without it, physicians will struggle to enhance patient care, achieve superior clinical outcomes, and streamline operations. Clinician effort will be vital. But without leadership capable of connecting the various parts of the healthcare system and evolving its method of reimbursement, the providers of care will encounter challenges too large to overcome.

Weaving technology together with operational excellence is no easy task, but it becomes possible with the right leadership. I saw this firsthand when a team of leaders in Kaiser Permanente applied predictive analytic technologies (a precursor to generative AI) in healthcare to save thousands of lives.

Accurately Predicting the Unexpected

The Permanente Medical Group's division of research stands as one of the nation's largest and most esteemed facilities. It has published groundbreaking clinical research on a vast range of medical challenges including cancer, vaccines, and heart disease. But its uniqueness lies in the ability to link research efforts with clinical practice.

Within this hub of innovation, Dr. Gabriel Escobar, a physician and researcher, led a critical investigation, backed by a robust team of IT and data analytics experts.

Their work focused on a perplexing issue that baffles physicians: why do some patients, seemingly on the mend, suddenly experience a severe decline in their clinical condition, necessitating urgent transfer to the intensive care unit for lifesaving care? The central question driving Dr. Escobar's study was whether modern technology could preemptively identify these at-risk patients before their condition worsened, thereby enabling timely interventions that could potentially save lives.

The team compiled data from 650,000 hospitalized patients, 20,000 of whom required urgent ICU transfer. Using this information, they developed an AI-based model capable of predicting which patients in a medical or surgical unit *today* are at the highest risk of requiring ICU care *tomorrow*. The researchers then tested the tool in the medical group's 20 hospitals throughout California.

Demonstrating that the model would work, medical-group leadership then implemented a dependable alert system for iPhones that would notify physicians when one of their patients was identified as "at risk." Leadership then obtained the commitment from the hospital-based physicians in each inpatient facility that they would respond immediately once alerted.

To reliably identify the patients most likely to decline in clinical status, the IT application used a wealth of information—including lab results, data from bedside monitoring devices, and vital signs input from the electronic healthcare record. While such a comprehensive analysis is beyond human capability, given the sheer volume of data and the need to assess thousands of patients daily, the computer system handled it with ease.

The tool's effectiveness was tested by implementing it in select inpatient facilities while other hospitals served as controls. This approach allowed researchers to rigorously assess its impact on clinical outcomes, particularly its ability to reduce mortality rates. In hospitals where the system was deployed, fewer patients experienced health declines that necessitated ICU transfers, underscoring the lifesaving potential of early intervention. Intriguingly, the study also revealed that patients who benefited from early interventions and avoided ICU stays had a significantly lower risk of dying (three to four times less) in the months following discharge compared to those who were admitted to the ICU and discharged after apparent recovery. This suggests that preventing health deterioration not only has immediate benefits but also contributes to longer-term patient survival.

These were huge findings. Conventionally, the discharge of both patient groups would have been considered a successful outcome in medical practice. Given that both sets of patients began with an equal risk of dying, the researchers had every reason to assume post-discharge mortality rates would be similar for both. But that assumption was proven wrong.

Encouraged by these compelling results, medical-group leaders rolled out the AI system across all 20-plus hospitals, effectively monitoring the health status of around 5,000 patients at any given moment. The AI system proved to be remarkably adept, pinpointing the 30 patients each day at "highest risk"—about one or two per hospital. For these patients, the mortality rate dropped 60 percent below expected outcomes, translating into thousands of lives saved annually.

The key lesson here extends beyond the power of innovative technology or the doctors' responsiveness to AI-generated alerts. It underscores the critical role of combining data-driven technological advancements with strong leadership. Without both of these elements, progress would stall and lives would be needlessly lost. When these forces align, however, tragedy is averted.

Technological Advancements in Patient Monitoring

Dr. Devi Shetty, a distinguished cardiac surgeon who once served as the personal physician to Mother Teresa, is at the forefront of healthcare transformation in India, skillfully combining modern technology, visionary leadership, and a commitment to systemness.

At his heart surgery hospitals, doctors achieve excellent clinical outcomes with help from innovative technologies that streamline processes, enhance communication, and synchronize the various components of the healthcare delivery system, all under the guidance of adept leadership.

A testament to his innovative approach is the advanced post-operative patient monitoring system he has implemented. This system is designed to identify subtle yet critical early indicators of potential complications, long before they escalate into severe threats. Central to his strategy is a patient-centric electronic health record system, bolstered by real-time data analytics and fluid communication channels, focusing on clinical (rather than financial) objectives.

When I went to visit his newest health system on Grand Cayman Island, three hours south of Miami, I was impressed that every patient admitted to his hospitals received a low-cost tablet, which not only provided them with continuous access to their medical records but also enabled direct communication with their healthcare team. This innovative use of technology ensures that vital patient information is always accessible, facilitating immediate and informed medical responses.

Central to Dr. Shetty's operation is a state-of-the-art monitoring hub, where large screens display live video feeds and vital patient data around the clock. This hub is staffed by experienced physicians who, thanks to Dr. Shetty's strategic use of global time zones, provide constant vigilance and rapid response to any signs of patient distress, no matter the time of day. By day, clinicians working in the Grand Cayman facility monitor the progress of patients across the night in India, and 12 hours later, the doctors in India make sure the patients 10,000 miles away are recovering safely.

Dr. Shetty's hospitals exemplify the powerful synergy between cutting-edge technology and human expertise, significantly improving response times to critical events. In his facilities, for example, it takes clinicians fewer than 10 minutes to act on potentially significant findings such as a slight increase in post-operative bleeding, an unexpected rise in pulse rate, or a drop in blood pressure or blood oxygen levels.

This rapid response contrasts sharply with the typical scenario in many US community hospitals, especially during nights and weekends, where it can take an hour or more to recognize and respond to these early warning signs of a looming health crisis. The result is that the surgeons in his hospitals in India achieve clinical outcomes that match the best in the United States at a cost of $1,800 per procedure (compared to an average price of $123,000 for heart bypass procedures in the United States).

Just like the work of Dr. Escobar and his team, the success of Dr. Shetty's methods goes beyond high-tech AI. It's about leaders creating a culture where fast and effective care is valued, and doctors, no matter how far apart geographically, work together on behalf of patients. This high-tech and high-touch solution not only saves lives and cuts down costs, but it also generates for clinicians a powerful sense of pride.

Outsmarting Dr. House

The TV series *House* captured the imagination of audiences by highlighting the remarkable intellect of a solitary doctor tackling complex medical mysteries. While entertaining, the narrative overlooked a fundamental truth about modern healthcare: no physician, regardless of individual talent or intellect, can match the collective capability of a diverse medical team supported by cutting-edge technology.

Tomorrow's healthcare landscape will be defined by more than individual acumen. Organizations will achieve the best outcomes through the synergy of dedicated medical professionals, empowered patients, and advanced AI tools.

Echoing the sentiments of Dr. Atul Gawande, a venerated figure in patient safety, medicine must move away from the romanticized image of the lone "cowboy" doctor, shifting toward a model reminiscent of Formula One pit crews. Just as these racing teams exhibit unmatched precision and teamwork to achieve their goals, American healthcare needs to adopt a similar approach—one where success is magnified by the ability of clinicians to work cohesively toward a common goal. How leaders accomplish this will be the remaining focus of part five.

PART FIVE | CHAPTER NINETEEN

LEADERSHIP: THE FOURTH PILLAR

Chapter 12 introduced three "pillars" necessary for securing the foundation of American healthcare's future: the integration of care, adopting prepayment (or "capitation") for medical services, and the emphasis on patient-centered technologies over profit-driven ones.

In this chapter, and throughout the rest of the book, we delve into a critical yet often overlooked aspect of healthcare transformation—leadership. It represents the final pillar necessary for navigating the challenges and leveraging the opportunities of Healthcare 4.0, ultimately leading to high-quality clinical outcomes and sustained affordability. Leadership is the linchpin for transitioning to value-based care in this new era.

Joel Barker, an early proponent of the concept of paradigm shifts, offers a compelling definition of leadership that resonates profoundly within the context of healthcare: "A leader is someone you would follow to a place you wouldn't go by yourself." This insight underscores the pivotal role of leaders in steering healthcare out of its current rut. To solve the immense challenges facing American healthcare, our nation needs leaders with the vision to see what others can't, the courage to take risks, and the skill to overcome big problems through brave actions.

Right now, such leadership is scarce in our nation. Instead of proactive leaders eager to confront and resolve the core issues plaguing healthcare, there's an abundance of intermediaries, content to apply superficial fixes to small problems rather than tackle the biggest ones. And they're quick to point their fingers when outcomes fall short. This surge in nonclinical middlemen, coupled with a shortage of clinical leaders, has fostered a culture of blame that permeates the entire US healthcare system. The purchasers of care blame the insurers for high costs and poor health. Insurers, in turn, blame the doctors. The providers blame patients, regulators, and fast-food companies. Patients blame their employers and the government. This blame game creates a vicious cycle of inaction, leaving the system's most pressing flaws and vulnerabilities unaddressed.

Of course, there are plenty of people in healthcare—CEOs, board chairs, medical-group presidents, and so on—with the power and ability to lead transformative change. But a combination of fear and insufficient skill limits their thinking and vision, causing them to make only small, incremental improvements.

As long as the healthcare solutions remain small, the consequences will grow bigger. Cautious solutions will not solve the huge problem of medical debt, which affects four in 10 Americans. Nor will they sufficiently enhance access to healthcare given that wait times have stretched to 26 days on average for patients in larger cities, with the even more substantial obstacles to access faced by those in rural areas. And without doubt, incremental steps will be inadequate to alleviate the pain of clinicians who have hit rock bottom—with nearly two-thirds reporting symptoms of burnout, leading to "higher rates of alcohol abuse and suicidal ideation, as well as increased medical errors and worse patient outcomes," according to the US Surgeon General.

A Wobbly Pillar

All over the country—in rural hospitals and big-city health systems, in clinics and corner offices—the people in charge of delivering excellent healthcare struggle to lead. No matter how hard they try, clinicians find it impossible to simultaneously improve quality, make care convenient, and contain costs.

Compounding these challenges is a "perfect storm" of escalating healthcare expenses, a critical shortage of healthcare professionals, and an increasing incidence of physician burnout. Together, these megatrends are plunging the healthcare system into turmoil.

Diving deeper into these challenges, recall that healthcare inflation during the pandemic was somewhat restrained. That's because many patients deferred non-urgent medical care due to fears of COVID-19 exposure in medical settings. However, the receding of the pandemic has led to a surge in demand for healthcare services. This resurgence in demand is negatively impacting insurers and placing additional financial burdens on American families, who are responsible for a large portion of their healthcare expenses. Complicating matters further, a significant percentage of nurses are contemplating leaving the profession, which is likely to compromise patient care and further drive costs upward. Nurses cite unrealistic job demands, hostile interactions with patients, and a lack of institutional support as their primary grievances. Additionally, a notable portion of physicians, including 32 percent of doctors in academic settings, are considering leaving their current positions within the next two years, driven by burnout and a sense of professional dissatisfaction.

Sensing control slipping through their fingers, independent physicians, hospital-based doctors, and physician groups are turning to private equity firms for greater negotiating power. Between 2010 and 2019, private equity's annual healthcare investments soared from $42 billion to $120 billion. These investments have resulted in higher reimbursement for participating clinicians, but they have also compromised clinician autonomy, led to unsafe cost-cutting measures, and undermined the ability of patients to afford medical care.

Given these massive challenges, it's logical to question why leaders would be willing to take on the risks associated with launching a healthcare revolution. Clinging to the prevailing middleman mindset would seem a safer and simpler choice.

While the status quo remains tempting for many, there are compelling reasons for leaders to take on the herculean task of transforming medicine.

- **Profit generation (opportunity).** Healthcare has been a lucrative business for middlemen. In an industry with over 80 "unicorns" (startup companies valued at over $1 billion), the majority of those enterprises offer point solutions for relatively minor problems. However, a far bigger prize awaits those who can solve the manifold issues of medical care delivery and health insurance. Capture even 5 percent of healthcare's total expenditures, and you'll claim more than $200 billion as your reward. The leading contenders capable of doing so include large medical groups, hospital systems, venture capitalists, and big corporations like Amazon, CVS, and Walmart.

• **Pain reduction (desperation).** Some of healthcare's biggest players are struggling badly. Hospital margins have eroded under the weight of inflation and the industry-wide shift to outpatient care. Medical groups, having suffered financial losses throughout the COVID-19 pandemic, are now forced to endure declining Medicare reimbursements (a trend that carried from 2023 to 2024). Community doctors are experiencing both declining revenues and diminishing workplace satisfaction. And so, if practically everyone is suffering, then perhaps now is the right time to challenge old assumptions and embrace a move for change. Whereas fee-for-service payments and fragmentation proved financially remunerative in the past, they are now causing great pains. Clinicians are spinning their legs ever faster on the care-delivery treadmill just to stay in place, which increases burnout and threatens economic security. A radical pivot may be the best (and perhaps only) chance for leaders to stop the bleeding.

• **Purpose and fulfillment (mission).** Though many healthcare players may be motivated by personal financial gain, medicine has long attracted individuals wanting to help others and save lives. A case in point came during the earliest days of the pandemic, when doctors and nurses selflessly put the health of patients ahead of their own lives. For many healthcare professionals, aligning their goal of excellence in patient care with their own well-being represents an opportunity to reignite the sense of purpose and mission that initially drew them to the medical field. Such alignment not only benefits patients but also reduces the intense burnout so many clinicians personally experience. Purpose can serve as an effective catalyst for physicians wanting to lead the necessary changes in healthcare. It also has the power to inspire like-minded clinicians to join and support this transformative journey.

Regardless of their motivations, all leaders face the challenge of where to begin in the quest to fix American healthcare. My recommendation: start by reframing the problem.

Redefining Leadership in Healthcare

In 1998, shortly after I was named CEO in Kaiser Permanente, I visited the Oregon Health Sciences center to keynote a conference on healthcare in the coming century. As I wandered the halls after my talk, a sign caught my attention.

In bold letters across the top, it read: "Cost. Access. Quality."

And below, in tiny font: "pick any two."

I found the message appropriate for the time, even if a bit sardonic. Back then, most administrators believed it was possible to improve in two of these areas but only at the expense of the third. Unfortunately, they were right. Even in the 1990s, medical practice lacked the knowledge, technology, and processes required to achieve excellence in all three areas.

Almost three decades later, this outdated mentality persists—despite radical scientific and technological advances, including evidence-based practices, deep data analytics, smartphones, telemedicine and, of course, artificial intelligence.

To healthcare's current leaders, the quandary of cost, quality, and access goes something like this: sure, it's possible to enhance the quality of (and access to) care by hiring a lot more people, but that will only drive unsustainable costs even higher. Likewise, it is possible to stem financial losses by laying off staff and restricting hours of operation, but that will only compromise clinical outcomes and patient satisfaction. As such, the goal of "value-based care," though frequently touted, remains more a distant dream than an impending reality for American medicine.

Healthcare leaders struggle to figure out how to connect all the disparate parts. They hesitate to move forward with change, dreading the resistance they will face when attempting to implement transformative strategies. They recognize how difficult it will be to win over the people who deliver care. Doctors dislike authority and prefer a flat, collegial structure. Healthcare pundits have jokingly described the effort of leading physicians as "herding cats." In contrast to industries that rely heavily on data, process, and collaborative decision-making, physicians prize their autonomy and view top-down leadership with great skepticism. Instead of seeing evidence-based methods as a means to enhance clinical outcomes, increase convenience, and reduce costs, many doctors dismiss them as restrictive or formulaic. "Cookbook medicine" they call it. Convincing medical professionals to adopt change involves not just a presentation of the current problems, but also a clear demonstration of the tangible benefits new approaches will bring.

For Healthcare 4.0 to succeed, the medical mindset will need to be different. Instead of perceiving quality, access, and cost as competing priorities, leaders in this next generation of medicine will need to devise and execute strategies that enhance affordability by simultaneously improving quality and access. The best approach to achieving all three is by keeping patients healthier. That means fewer chronic diseases, reduced complications from the ones patients already have, and greater empowerment of patients in the provision of medical care. And the best way to accomplish all these parts will be to embrace generative AI. Without doing so, leaders will find themselves trapped in the eras of Healthcare 2.0 and 3.0, unable to provide the value clinicians and patients expect. Just as space shuttles can't escape the pull of gravity without thruster rockets, medicine won't escape its current inertia without the power of generative AI technology.

The Anatomy of Healthcare Leadership

As we delve deeper into the qualities necessary for transformative healthcare leadership, three core "anatomical structures" stand out: the heart, the brain, and the spine. Though not part of the traditional curriculum in medical or nursing schools, mastering this anatomy is pivotal for the future of medicine. To achieve excellence in healthcare, leaders must possess the ability to change people's minds, generate emotion and passion, and maintain courage in the face of adversity.

- **The brain.** Medical students are selected based on standardized tests, which aim to measure intelligence and problem-solving abilities. Therefore, leaders who wish to drive change in medical practice must lead with logic—presenting a clear vision, offering sound arguments, and engaging in intellectual debate. In addition, they must listen to, and work alongside, clinicians, helping them weigh the pros and cons of change before mandating it. And, finally, they must avoid the mistake of thinking the brain is the only (or even most important) anatomic structure necessary to connect with others.
- **The heart.** The mind is compelled by logic, but the heart is moved by emotion, passion, and the power of story. Leaders who tell strong narratives and convey patient testimonies are more successful in helping people overcome the fear of change. Passion is equally important because no one will care how much a leader knows unless they know how much the leader cares. When leaders express a sincere desire to help others and save lives, they form a powerful bond with clinicians. Reconnecting doctors and nurses with a higher sense of purpose has the power to touch the heart in ways no logical argument ever could.
- **The spine.** Even when people are convinced that change is important, they still need the courage to act. Leaders must demonstrate both resolve and resilience during the painful transition process. Not surprisingly, the most common concern I hear from future leaders is, "But if I make those changes, people will push back." I tell them, "If you're not encountering resistance, you're not leading." Helping people move forward in the face of uncertainty is a critical skill. A strong spine supports the leader in hard times and gives followers greater confidence that the future will be better than the present.

Embodying these leadership traits will go a long way toward sparking the transformation. But desire, alone, won't deliver success to the medical system. The next chapter shifts focus from the will to lead to the practicalities of implementing change. To help leaders wanting to drive transformative solutions, we will explores how to bridge the current gap, turning aspirations and insights into concrete actions and effective strategies, powerful enough to reshape the entire healthcare system.

PART FIVE | CHAPTER TWENTY

POLE POSITION

For all the remarkable opportunities generative AI offers American healthcare, hope for transformative change hinges on the human element above all else.

The story of Ernest Shackleton, an early 20th-century explorer, exemplifies the fortitude needed to navigate extreme risk—and it demonstrates the difference exceptional leadership can make.

Having already reached the South Pole in 1910, the captain understood his next voyage would be far more challenging and potentially deadly. In an era that would come to define adventure and discovery, Shackleton hoped to cross the entire continent of Antarctica, from one end to the other, *over* the South Pole.

Legend has it, Shackleton placed posters all throughout London to recruit his crew, warning that the expedition would be dangerous and filled with hardship. It took two years to raise the necessary funds, hire 56 sailors, and purchase the requisite 59 dogs he would depend on for the 1,800-mile trek across the frozen tundra. With all the supplies in place, two boats headed out of port from Plymouth, England, in early fall 1914.

Half the crew was aboard each ship. *Endurance* carried the main crew to the north side of the continent in the Weddell Sea. The *Aurora* took a group of sailors to the opposite side of Antarctica, directly in line with the landing spot of the first boat, ready to take the sailors home after their march across the pole. Once ashore, the crew upon the second boat would harness the dog sleds and travel inland toward the South Pole, as far as it could, leaving food and fuel supplies for the first group as it completed the second half of its transcontinental expedition.

For the endeavor, Shackelton selected a diverse crew with eccentric interests. Unlike other captains of the time, he distributed the daily chores equally among the seamen, officers, and scientists. And different from his contemporaries, Shackelton socialized with everyone on board the ship, playing games, singing songs, and joking merrily.

Second in command was the explorer Frank Wild who had accompanied the captain on his previous journey to the South Pole. Though their last journey was a failure in the eyes of many—arriving at the pole behind a competing expedition—Wild told anyone who would listen about the crew's thrilling journey. He'd recounted an instance when he, himself, had fallen desperately ill, and it was Shackleton who offered Wild his allotted biscuit for the day. Wild wrote in his diary, "All the money that was ever minted would not have bought that biscuit and the remembrance of that sacrifice will never leave me."

As *Endurance* set out across the Weddell Sea, conditions worsened. By mid-January, the vessel was frozen solid in an ice floe. For the next five weeks, the crew engaged in daily routines as though departure was imminent. Assignments included caring for the dogs, repairing equipment, ensuring the lifeboats were ready, and melting snow to fill water containers. One of the ship's surgeons wrote that Shackleton "did not rage at all or show outwardly the slightest sign of disappointment," and instead, "He told us simply and calmly that we must winter in the Pack: explained its dangers and possibilities: never lost his optimism and prepared for winter."

By the end of February, the weather had become more frigid, and it was clear that the ship would remain trapped in the ice at least until September, when spring in the Southern Hemisphere arrived. It was a brutal winter. Rations thinned out, as did the men. As the days warmed, slowly the ice began to shift. But rather than dislodging the ship, the movements exerted extreme pressure on the hull. Water rushed in. On October 24, 1915, Shackleton ordered the crew to take everything they could from the ship and abandon the wreck. A little less than a month later, the ship sank.

For six months, the crew rode the ice floes, hoping they would drift to safe landing, but fate was against them. The ice floe broke in half. And with civilization nowhere in sight, Shackleton ordered the crew onto the lifeboats. After five exhausting days at sea, the three small crafts landed at Elephant Island, 346 miles and 497 days from where and when they began.

Conditions were brutal, but Shackleton never stopped thinking about the crew. He gave his mittens to a photographer who'd lost his pair on the journey. As a result, Shackleton suffered frostbite on his fingers.

Elephant Island wasn't a likely place for rescue, so the captain decided to make an open-boat journey to the South Georgia whaling station where help might be found. Shackleton picked a crew of five and headed out with only four weeks of supplies. He accepted that if the boat didn't reach its destination by that time, he and the others would already be dead. Two weeks later, they landed on the rugged shore. Shackleton and two men climbed for 36 straight hours, scaling the intervening mountain with its dangerous, rocky terrain.

On May 20, 1916, they reached shelter. When the three crewmen walked into the whaling station, the manager turned to the bearded man and asked, "Who the hell are you?"

The man replied, "I'm Shackleton." In utter disbelief, the manager turned back around and wept, having long assumed the expedition was lost to the depths.

From the station, Shackleton immediately sent a boat to the other side of the island to pick up the remaining three members of his rescue party and contemplated how he would reach the other 22 sailors from the Endeavor. It would take him four attempts, but on August 30 of that year, he arrived, four and a half months after he had left them to seek help. Incredibly, he brought home all 27 of the men who had sailed on the Endeavor with him.

Five years later, in 1921, he launched another expedition to Antarctica. As unbelievable as it might seem, eight members of his previous crew signed on to accompany him despite the perils of the previous expedition.

Along the way, Shackleton suffered a heart attack and died in his bunk. Frank Wild, his number two, steered the ship toward the frozen coast, but once again couldn't penetrate the floes. He pointed the ship north and headed home, never to return.

Ernest Shackleton's remarkable and arduous journey across Antarctica is a tale of extraordinary leadership, resilience, and strategic acumen. Despite his failure to complete the expedition, this narrative provides insights into how healthcare leaders can best navigate the complexities of modern medicine in the era of Healthcare 4.0. Among the lessons for medical leaders:

- Building a unified team is essential. Shackleton spent months planning the journey, assembling a diverse crew, and finalizing the detailed logistics for the cross-continental trek. In Healthcare 4.0, leaders must similarly employ strategic vision and meticulous planning to integrate new technologies, manage resources, and navigate the evolving healthcare landscape.
- Instilling trust and allaying fears are critical. The uncertainties Shackleton faced are akin to the challenges of transforming healthcare. Leaders must inspire confidence, persuading healthcare professionals of the benefits of new reimbursement models and technologies, even if it means adjusting long-established practices and ceding some of their autonomy to do what is best for the group.
- Steadfast leadership is nonnegotiable. Shackleton's unwavering resolve in the face of adversity is a model for healthcare leaders venturing into new territories. Embracing innovative care methods and empowering patients to take charge of their health will require courage and persistence to overcome inevitable obstacles.
- The leader's integrity is the foundation of success. Throughout the ordeal, Shackleton always maintained a strong focus on the welfare of his crew. They responded with total confidence that he'd put their needs ahead of his own. Clinicians will sacrifice almost anything for their patients, but they are wary of those who take on leadership roles for personal benefit. Top-down authority doesn't succeed in times of difficult change. Clinicians will not accept the risks of embracing GenAI or capitation if they doubt the leader's motivation and commitment.

***

Leadership and administration, often conflated in healthcare, serve distinct functions. Administrators do what is expected and necessary to keep healthcare organizations running. They ensure operational continuity and attend to their requisite legal, financial, and logistic responsibilities.

Leaders, by contrast, make things happen that otherwise would not. Great leaders move forward with assurance, knowing that once the destination is reached, no one will want to go back to where the organization started. They do this by creating a vision, aligning people around it, and giving them the confidence needed to move forward.

Often what's missing in times of stagnant leadership is the energy to get the change process started. In the realm of science, initiating change demands a greater exertion of effort compared to maintaining momentum once it's established. This principle holds true for leaders facing the formidable task of igniting transformative change within an entrenched healthcare system. The concept of "activation energy" in chemistry—a term denoting the minimum energy necessary to start a reaction—aptly mirrors the initial push required to shift healthcare from its current state toward a more innovative and patient-centered future.

Picture a colossal boulder nestled within a crater, representing the healthcare system's status quo. The biggest challenge lies not in the force needed to propel the huge rock forward once it gains momentum, but in the Herculean effort required to dislodge the boulder from its resting place. Each attempt to push it over the crater's rim is met with resistance, akin to the current inertia within healthcare, making the initial movement the most dangerous and arduous phase of transformation.

The introduction of ChatGPT and other generative AI tools serve as a catalyst in this scenario, effectively lowering the metaphorical crater walls and reducing the requisite activation energy. These technological advancements, while potent, will not single-handedly propel the system forward. They will require the complement of visionary leadership to realize their potential. It is the synergy of innovative technology and dynamic leadership that promises to finally push the boulder of healthcare transformation beyond its long-standing barriers, setting it in motion toward a future of enhanced care and improved outcomes. The next chapter explores an effective method to do so.

PART FIVE | CHAPTER TWENTY-ONE

LEADERSHIP: FROM A TO G

In healthcare, where transformation centers on the collective will of practitioners, leadership faces a difficult dilemma. The journey toward change in medicine demands a pace that neither exceeds the capacity of the organization's members nor stalls out. The art of transformational leadership lies in stretching the system's capabilities without fracturing the spirit of its people.

Imagine yourself the leader of a large healthcare organization. You can clearly visualize a future where clinicians and staff lead the nation in quality, accessibility, and cost-effectiveness. You see a horizon, two maybe three years out, glimmering with the promise of GPT-6 (whatever it'll be called) and the seamless integrations of wearable tech, electronic health records, and AI-powered voice commands. Despite your team's commendable clinical performance, the chasm between the current state and the pinnacle of what's possible yawns wide.

In recent years, your patient and clinician satisfaction scores have waned, financial pressures are mounting, and the threat of reduced reimbursement looms as insurance-network exclusions threaten your organization's stability.

Convinced that value-based care, bolstered by the judicious application of generative AI, is the key to rising above these challenges, you unveil your vision at the quarterly meeting to the entire organization. There, you announce a bold plan to move from the transactional fee-for-service model to a capitated, transformational system of care that promises to reward the entire medical group for collective achievement. Knowing you're doing what's right for the health system and its patients, you brace for raucous applause.

Instead, your grand strategy is met with palpable silence. What went wrong?

The quiet resistance that meets your announcement is not a rejection of your vision but a reflection of deep-seated fears and uncertainties. The human psyche is wired to weigh losses more heavily than gains, a principle that holds true especially in healthcare—a risk-adverse profession. The potential downsides of these financial changes loom larger in the minds of clinicians than the long-term benefits of your plan. Moreover, a pervasive distrust of leadership's intentions and concerns about fairness and transparency in the new system exacerbate the resistance. Your strategy, while forward-thinking, has inadvertently bypassed the crucial step of aligning people's perceptions and emotions with the proposed path forward.

To navigate this impasse, it's imperative to recognize that visionary leadership extends beyond the mere presentation of a plan. As the last chapter pointed out, it requires deep engagement with the hearts and minds of those you aim to lead—addressing their fears while building trust through clarity and empathy. The journey to transformative change in healthcare is about people. To help them move forward, you'll need to understand and address the worries that hold them back.

If you had sat among the audience during the presentation and listened to comments whispered between colleagues, you'd have overheard more than a dozen concerns: *If capitation fails, will I be able to pay my mortgage and send my kids to college? What if generative AI makes an error, will I be held responsible? Why should we do this if no one else in the medical community is making the change? Will I have to work more nights and weekends? Will I have to work longer each day? Will I ever see my family again? Can I trust leadership this time or is this just another bait and switch? Am I a fool for signing on? Will this new system be fair?* The list is endless.

Your tendency—and that of many leaders—might be to impose your will and forge ahead, propelled by the urgency of your mission. However, the path to transformative success is paved with patience, dialogue, and understanding. This realization—that there's a series of tasks that must be completed to lead change—led me to create the "A to G model," a structured approach to transforming healthcare.

While far from an exhaustive list, it offers a robust framework to embark on the arduous journey healthcare leaders face today.

The A to G Model

The quest to transform American healthcare into a more integrated and efficient system necessitates more than just individual effort or incremental change. The sheer scale of change required transcends the capabilities of solo practitioners or small groups, who lack the resources to implement operational efficiencies and achieve economies of scale. Medical groups and large healthcare systems, with their broader capabilities and reach, are the entities best positioned to blaze the trail. Once they chart the course, physicians in communities nationwide can adopt these transformative tools, unite, and follow their lead.

The transition from traditional, smaller-scale practices to an integrated and efficient healthcare system—capable of embracing innovative financial models and harnessing modern technology—represents a monumental shift in the practice of medicine. However, achieving scale is merely a starting point and not a strategy in itself. The real work lies in redesigning the delivery of medical care and securing the dedication of those tasked with executing the plan.

This is where the A to G model comes into play. It is designed to guide this extensive transformation, not just within healthcare but in any industry facing the daunting task of comprehensive change. This model outlines a strategic approach to achieving excellence by detailing the steps necessary for organizations to adapt and thrive in an evolving landscape. Its principles are universal, providing a roadmap for leaders across all sectors looking to steer their organizations through the complexities of transformation.

Each letter of the A to G mnemonic in this chapter addresses one or more fears people will encounter along the way. The order is alphabetic, not temporal. The medical examples provided within are generic. The details will vary based on the structure of the organization (e.g., a medical group versus hospital staff model versus health system), its geography (city, suburban, or rural), and the starting point (single specialty, multi-specialty, or comprehensive care, including both clinicians from a broad range of disciplines and one or more hospitals).

But despite these variations, skipping any of these seven steps is a prescription for failure in every setting.

"A" Stands for Aspirational Vision

For leaders, it's impossible to win over the minds of colleagues unless you connect with their hearts. An aspirational vision serves not just as a destination but as a call to action, compelling individuals to commit, to dare, and to dream.

Consider the story of Ernest Shackleton whose call to adventure was not laden with promises of wealth but with the allure of achieving the extraordinary. It was this vision of a remarkable endeavor that brought together a crew eager to accomplish something greater than themselves. This same kind of drive can be found in the hearts of medical students, fueled by a noble purpose. Unfortunately, once the constraints of a faltering healthcare system take hold, many find their flame is dimmed. But, still, the embers glow deep inside them. As such, the potential to rekindle this passion lies with visionary leaders. It is a leader's job to inspire.

Importantly, an aspirational vision must also be grounded in achievable realities, making it not a mere dream but a palpable goal. To motivate, it should extend beyond personal ambition to encapsulate the very essence of healthcare's impact: lives saved, patients benefited by convenience, and financial burdens eased. These visions come alive when explained through the lens of real-life people—stories that resonate with the heart and soul of healthcare professionals.

Doctors appreciate stories of real patients who've overcome chronic pain thanks to a physician's help. They are touched to hear of grandparents who've attended graduations and weddings they never thought possible. They are moved by the narrative of a single mother for whom healthcare is no longer a logistic nightmare, and a young couple facing severe health challenges without the fear of financial ruin. For clinicians, making such positive outcomes a reality is a goal worth pursuing. Although enhancing a hospital's financial health and adhering to regulatory mandates are critical administrative objectives, they do not inspire physicians. And these types of goals pale in comparison to improving lives. Such narratives have the power to inspire clinicians to embrace risks and innovate boldly.

An aspirational vision need not captivate everyone, but if it resonates deeply with a significant minority, it can build collective momentum. Psychological research demonstrates that a committed 25 to 30 percent of a group is a sufficient tipping point for widespread change.

Throughout history, iconic leaders have understood the power of aspirational vision to affect change. This ability was epitomized by Martin Luther King Jr. in his "I Have a Dream" speech. King's words did not promise the impossible eradication of hatred or even prejudice, but they painted a picture of a future filled with hope and unity.

"Right there in Alabama," he said, "little Black boys and Black girls will be able to join hands with little white boys and white girls as sisters and brothers," a vision both bold and within the realm of possibility as evidenced today by the camaraderie of youth sports across the nation.

Aspirational visions are like distant, majestic peaks—visible destinations that inspire people to march forward even when the path ahead is difficult or uncertain. And once individuals believe that what is being asked is possible, their commitment grows.

Shackleton's crew was driven by the prospect of pioneering an icy wilderness. They knew how hard it would be, but they also believed they could be successful. Similarly, healthcare professionals today are drawn to the noble ideals of medicine: advancing health and leveraging technology to alleviate suffering. Once leaders help them see how innovations like ChatGPT will facilitate this process and the positive impact it will have on people's lives, a once-distant dream edges closer to reality.

"B" Is for Behaviors

Behaviors, the tangible expressions of commitment, are the bedrock upon which the aspirations of Healthcare 4.0 rest. Success in this new era in medicine requires more than visionary thinking. It also demands clear, actionable changes from every participant in the healthcare continuum.

The tale of Shackleton's expedition is instructive here, illustrating the power of clear expectations. His crew was not lured by vague promises nor propelled by unclear expectations. The captain provided a candid outline of the challenges ahead and detailed the specific roles each member of the crew would play, focusing on equal distribution of tasks. Everyone understood exactly what was required to melt snow for water, prepare meals for a crew of 27, repair and maintain a boat, and care for 59 dogs. This level of clarity is what leaders must strive for when guiding their teams through the complexities of technological integration and operational innovation.

Behaviors are concrete and observable, not mere attitudes or platitudes. Many clinicians have been burned by leaders who spoke of working "smarter, not harder," only to find themselves working harder and longer under the new strategy. This discrepancy—between a leaders' promises and the reality of their implementations—erodes trust. No clinician will fall for such vague assurances twice.

Setting clear expectations is the cornerstone of fostering behavioral change. It's crucial to outline the daily behaviors and choices that collectively drive transformation, ensuring individuals understand that the demands on them will be manageable. It is the only way to address people's anxieties.

When it comes to embracing change, a common apprehension among doctors is the fear of overwhelming demands. For instance, the notion of teaching patients to input data into ChatGPT might seem daunting, conjuring images of hours added to an already packed schedule. However, when the actual expectation is straightforward—as in directing patients to health education resources or providing a handout with instructions for an online tutorial—people perceive the task as doable, requiring less than a minute per patient.

Setting clear expectations can ease a range of concerns. For example, doctors might initially dread the frequent interruptions and urgent patient alerts generated by AI monitoring. However, anxieties about patient care responsibilities will lessen once physicians understand that they will be given a two-hour window to respond during the day (and that a dedicated call center will handle emergency alerts). Knowing that a specialized team of doctors and nurses will address urgent communications overnight will alleviate concerns about disrupted sleep.

By setting clear expectations around specific behaviors, leaders can help clinicians value AI's potential to enhance care while overcoming their concerns that empowering patients will make the doctor's day more difficult (and their nights and weekends impossible). When everyone knows the rules and follows them, leaders gain commitment and group excellence grows.

Fairness, too, plays a crucial role in defining and sustaining new behaviors. Just as Shackleton made it clear that everyone would be expected to do their part—from the lowest ranking member of the crew to the most senior officers—healthcare leaders must ensure that expectations are balanced and equitable, both within and across departments. In the absence of well-defined expectations, clinicians have no choice but to rely on guesswork, resulting in inconsistent performance and leading everyone to the perception that they are contributing more than anyone else.

How highly people value fairness can be observed in what behavioral economists call the "ultimatum game." In it, two participants sitting in different rooms must decide how to split a sum, usually $100. One proposes the split, and the other either accepts or rejects it. If rejected, both get nothing. Despite economic logic suggesting any non-zero offer should be accepted, people usually reject splits that seem unfair, especially those that fail to reward them with at least 25 percent of the total. This underscores a fundamental human trait: people value fairness as strongly as financial gain.

Leaders will need to address concerns around fairness head on at the start of Healthcare 4.0 as job expectations evolve and the method of allocating dollars shifts. Clarity around expected behavioral changes will be essential as individual autonomy for care delivery morphs into new opportunities to provide superior medical care.

"C" Is for Context

In many industries, leaders invoke the concept of a "burning platform" to spark change, presenting their organizations with a crisis that demands immediate action. This tactic can galvanize people when the threat is palpable and urgent. For example, in Shackleton's harrowing adventure, the visible crisis of a ship trapped in ice required immediate, decisive action. That situation, clear and urgent to all, motivated everyone to go the extra mile.

Indeed, in turbulent waters, leaders must be vigilant, responsive, and prepared to lead their teams, drawing on the strength of a shared vision and the collective resolve to navigate through crises. But a burning platform's effectiveness wanes considerably once the crisis passes. Trying to invoke a new one just to drive performance will lead to crisis fatigue, a state all too familiar in the American healthcare landscape. In medicine, the stakes are perpetually high, which is why change is best accomplished through strategic thinking and clearly defined tactics.

Doctors and nurses lose trust when leaders invoke a false sense of urgency as the imperative for change. This underscores the importance of context. In contrast to an aspirational vision, this part of the A to G model is all about delivering the facts. These help people understand their situation, logically and analytically, offering details that help them to dispassionately assess the risks and opportunities in healthcare's ever-shifting landscape.

Explaining context is how leaders show respect for the intelligence of doctors and makes them feel valued. People may disagree with a new direction, but with context, at least they understand why the leader believes it is the best option available.

In healthcare, change doesn't occur in isolation. It is influenced by broader economic, technological, and social shifts. The complexities of healthcare's evolution, such as the advent of generative AI, the impact of retail giants, and the growing empowerment of patients, require time to grasp and patience to explain. For leaders, the economic landscape of healthcare underscores the urgent need for change and, for clinicians, highlights the benefits of transformation: half a nation struggling with medical expenses, a national debt exceeding the country's GDP, rising medical inflation outpacing wages, healthcare costs set to grow by an additional $3 trillion by 2031, and 90 million Americans relying on Medicaid—all paint a clear picture of an imminent financial crisis in healthcare.

Doctors enjoy flexing their intellectual muscle and engaging in debate. For this reason, leaders will be challenged in their interpretations of "context." When presented with leadership's version of "why," colleagues will ask: "Why not just raise prices instead of changing the entire reimbursement model?" "Why not sell to private equity to increase our leverage against insurers?" "If we take on more financial risk, what happens if there's another viral pandemic?" "What happens if Congress bans ChatGPT or OpenAI folds?"

Leaders need to be ready to address these legitimate concerns. Doing so requires thorough preparation. Presenting clear, fact-based responses will reinforce the credibility of the proposed direction. The concept of Black Swan events, introduced by Nassim Taleb, underscores the unpredictability and significant impact of rare occurrences. Although it's impossible to prepare for every unforeseen event, leaders are tasked with steering through challenges that are predictable based on existing trends and data. Only by showcasing their capability to manage these known issues can leaders inspire the necessary level of commitment from clinicians for meaningful change.

"D" Is for Data

Physicians are scientists. And when confronted with the possibility of doing anything new, they insist on having the numbers to validate its effectiveness before they commit. At the same time, almost all doctors believe they are practicing at the top of their specialty. And, of course, that's not mathematically possible. For both of these obstacles, data helps medical professionals more accurately assess their performance and understand possible improvements.

Sharing comparative data on clinical outcomes within any single department is one way to highlight potential opportunities. Of course, when the numbers aren't personally favorable, the first reaction of people is to assume the data are flawed or that an underperforming doctor is caring for the sickest or most demanding patients, thus skewing the numbers. Rarely is this the case.

Data serves as a powerful catalyst for change when presented effectively. Showcasing benchmarks and internal comparisons helps to underscore not just where gaps exist but also the potential for improvement. An educational process, rather than a punitive one, shifts a defensive response to a proactive search for solutions.

And once a transformation effort is launched, data will be essential to measure progress and identify new opportunities. Anticipation and preparation are vital to effectively using data. Leaders need to determine in advance what information will be distributed on a weekly or monthly basis, and how it will be used. More importantly, they must know what they will do if results fall short of the goal. If quality outcomes or patient satisfaction results don't meet expectations and leaders fail to act, the message they send to clinicians is clear: the strategic plan is unimportant. Once that nonchalance becomes embedded in an organization's culture, the ship will begin to sink.

Shackleton based his actions on data. Knowing the distance to monitoring stations and the quantity of the remaining supplies, helped keep his men alive. As a result, the crew understood and accepted his decisions as logical, not idiosyncratic. The same is vital in helping clinicians understand current performance and the areas of greatest opportunity for the future.

As an example, when doctors treat patients with headaches, there's a notable variance in the frequency with which they order brain scans—differing as much as fourfold among physicians treating similar cases. This discrepancy suggests that some are ordering too many scans, while others too few. A thorough review of patient outcomes in comparable cases, based on whether a radiological study was performed, provides a more objective basis for ordering brain scans than a doctor's intuition or anecdotal experience.

In times of transformation, data points shine a light on exemplary practices, offering a platform for all clinicians to learn from and elevate their own standards of care.

"E" Is for Engagement.

Of the seven parts to this model, engagement is the most important. That's because no one will care how much you know until they know how much you care.

Implementing change in healthcare requires that leaders meet personally with individuals and with groups of medical care providers.

There is no other way to develop the trust needed and make sure your vision and ideas are understood.

Doctors, burdened by the daily sprint of medical practice and fearful of committing errors that could kill a patient, will dread the discomfort that change might bring, both for their patients and themselves. Those who've had a previous experience of feeling misled by leadership will be even more apprehensive about new initiatives and reluctant to endorse yet another plan that might not succeed. Their past makes them wary of championing a failing cause and, thus, appearing inept or foolish to their peers.

Trust in leadership occurs when words match actions over time. If your motivation is self-serving and not in the best interest of the people you lead or the patients they serve, their trust will erode. And until leaders demonstrate impeccable integrity and reliability over time, those asked to change will withhold their trust.

The only way to convince others of your sincerity and authenticity is through consistent action and engagement. Shackleton was a model of this.

He engaged with his crew on a daily basis and demonstrated great consistency with his actions. Recall that Shackleton didn't isolate himself from the crew. Instead, he actively participated in the evening's festivities. He also gave up his day's rations for his second in command and gave his gloves to the photographer who had lost his. And when all 27 members of his crew were hopelessly stranded, he led the expedition to find help, climbing a cragged mountain for more than a day, then making four attempts at rescue before achieving success. It was no surprise that eight crew members signed on for his next voyage despite their near-death experience.

The story of Shackleton has become a case study in leadership, in part because of the extremes to which he went. The rest of us won't be capable of matching it, but we all can learn from it. More than anything, we as leaders can demonstrate to the people who follow us how much they matter. And we can do this every day, using both our words and deeds.

Colin Powell, one of the greatest military generals in US history, was renowned for never eating until everyone under his command had received their food. That's a level of gratitude and commitment all leaders can emulate. Too often, CEOs see themselves as entitled to push to the head of the line. They need to remember that everything they do is observed and graded by those who follow. When healthcare leaders take extra privileges for themselves or fail to provide excellent quality and service to their patients, clinicians won't follow them regardless of the brilliance of their ideas.

Remember that no one will be more committed to change or more likely to encourage others to join in the effort than you are as the leader. Engagement, not title, generates respect and leads to commitment.

"F" Is for Faculty

Faculty, a term traditionally reserved for academic staff at universities, here is reimagined to describe the core team surrounding a healthcare CEO. It refers to the leader's direct reports and other trusted members of the leadership team. Their main task is to provide the leader with expertise, assist with strategy, and help lead the change process.

If the goal is to use technologies like ChatGPT to empower patients, the faculty will provide expertise in a diverse range of areas: IT, finance, operational improvements, regulatory requirements, clinical quality, and patient education.

A trusted faculty is vital because leaders, even the most visionary and strategic, have blind spots. Those leaders who accept their own limitations are willing to seek out strong individuals who complement their skills and offset their weaknesses. These leaders must encourage team members to challenge their opinions.

For Shackleton, Frank Wild was that person. He was the glue that kept the operational pieces together day after day. He was the equivalent of both a chief operating and a chief people officer. When Shackleton wasn't present, he maintained the esprit de corps, told stories to establish the culture, and identified problems that needed attention. And when Shackleton died, Wild continued the voyage to the best of his ability and then ensured that the entire crew returned to England safely.

As healthcare shifts from traditional fee-for-service models to capitated systems, from fragmented care to integrated services, and from cost-inflating technologies to efficiency-driving tools, the faculty's importance and responsibilities will grow.

Implementing each of these changes is challenging in its own right. Combined, they demand a highly effective team. Leadership can often feel like a relentless and solitary path. Sharing the journey with a motivated and trustworthy team makes it more enjoyable and rewarding.

"G" Is for Governance.

Individual doctors who work in their own offices answer no one. Larger organizations (and even smaller, integrated medical groups) can't operate this way. They need a structure for making decisions, allocating resources, and measuring performance. Without these elements, any vision for the future is likely to become a mirage.

Inside larger health organizations, governance has three parts. All are important.

> 1. **Formal structure.** Usually, there is a board or equivalent oversight group that must affirm the organization's direction, along with key parts of the operative and financial plan. Frequently, the people in the medical group or health system perceive the organization chart as the sole governance structure. But new leaders soon realize that although board members have an important fiduciary responsibility, the informal structure is equally important in implementing transformational change.
>
> 2. **Informal structure.** This aspect of governance includes the leaders without a high-ranking title. These are "influencers" who colleagues look to before deciding whether they will embrace change. Informal leaders are powerful and vocal forces, capable of driving or inhibiting change. Before meeting with the large group, leaders are wise to meet one-on-one with these individuals and garner their support.
>
> 3. **Incentive structure.** Finally, most organizations use financial incentives to motivate behavior. Leaders tend to view these "carrots

and sticks" as the most effective tools, but rarely is that the case. Financial incentives for performance are powerful drivers of change. But, in healthcare, they rarely lead to the outcomes desired. Unintended consequences almost always are the result. As an example of this problem, I had a conversation with a leader from a medical group who implemented a compensation model for gastroenterologists based on the volume of colonoscopies performed. Traditionally, if a potentially precancerous polyp was discovered during a screening, the physician would remove it immediately, assuming there were no medical contradictions. However, after the shift to volume-based compensation, these physicians began scheduling a second colonoscopy for polyp removal instead of addressing it during the initial procedure. This change, driven by the new payment structure, led to lower quality care, added inconvenience for patients, and increased healthcare costs due to the unnecessary duplication of procedures.

Shackleton didn't use financial incentives to drive performance. Instead, he carefully selected individuals whom he thought would rise to the occasion when challenges arose. He focused on ways to maximize group performance, never singling out a superstar or pitting one member of the crew against another. Regardless of the circumstance, playing on a winning team improves clinician satisfaction and increases the level of fulfillment for all.

There are no shortcuts when implementing effective changes in clinical practice. The purpose of the A to G model is to remind leaders of all the steps needed for success. Skip a step and the initiative will fail. Fail to provide an aspirational vision and physicians won't hear the context, or care about the behaviors and data. Fail to engage as a leader or to achieve a cohesive faculty, and success will prove illusive.

As logical as the A to G model is, one final element proves essential for success, and that is serendipity. This book's final chapter looks at this variable, differentiates it from luck, and explains what people can do to embrace it with the highest probability of success.

PART FIVE | CHAPTER TWENTY-TWO

SEIZING SERENDIPITY

In the annals of medical innovation, serendipity has played a quiet but crucial role, transforming chance encounters and unexpected events into lifesaving discoveries. Again and again, some of history's most significant medical breakthroughs have arisen not solely from the rigors of research and deliberate innovation, but from serendipity's gentle nudge. This phenomenon, often overlooked, has been the silent ally of progress, guiding the hands of researchers and clinicians and reshaping modern medicine.

Consider the discovery of penicillin by Alexander Fleming, a classic tale of serendipity in action. In 1928, Fleming stumbled upon this medical milestone when he noticed that a mold, later identified as *penicillium notatum*, had accidentally contaminated one of his staphylococcus bacteria cultures. Around the mold, there was a clear ring where the bacteria could not grow. This chance discovery could have been dismissed as a mere laboratory mishap. In fact, it's likely that another scientist in Fleming's lab would have simply washed away the "contaminated" dish without a second thought. Instead, the mold caught Fleming's attention. He saw potential in the unexpected, leading to the development of the world's first antibiotic. This "happy accident" would go on to save millions of lives and forever change the course of medicine.

A similar story of chance accompanied a remarkable discovery made by Wilhelm Conrad Roentgen in 1895. During his experiments with cathode rays, Roentgen observed an unexpected glow on a chemically coated screen nearby. Curious as to what it could mean, he looked closer, and closer, ultimately leading him to identify a new type of ray.

He named it the "x-ray." As in Fleming's lab, this serendipitous observation could have been easily dismissed or overlooked, but Roentgen recognized the significance. And in doing so, he ushered in a new era in medical diagnostics through non-invasive internal examinations of the human body.

A word of caution: in thinking about these historical discoveries, don't attribute progress to dumb luck. While serendipity may present the initial spark, it is the prepared mind, ready to perceive and act upon unforeseen possibilities, that truly drives innovation. The ability and willingness to seize an opportunity is what transforms serendipity from an accidental or arbitrary occurrence into a groundbreaking innovation.

The act of seizing serendipity was vividly illustrated in the rapid development of COVID-19 vaccines in 2020. Prior to the pandemic, scientists had been exploring mRNA technology for various applications, absent a specific focus on coronaviruses and without any luck. However, when COVID-19 emerged as a global threat, researchers took the opportunity to quickly pivot and apply their existing knowledge toward developing an effective vaccine in record time.

Time and again, revolutionary change happens when events out of people's control intersect with individuals who recognize opportunity and seize the potential. This combination applies not just to medicine. Throughout my career, I have encountered unexpected opportunities that have altered my life for the better. I've learned that when these opportunities arise, you must be ready to seize them.

My path to medicine and healthcare leadership were both shaped by serendipity and a willingness to embrace unforeseen chances. During my college years, for instance, I planned to become a university professor. However, when my mentor was denied tenure for political reasons, I, in my naivete, chose medical school instead, believing matters of life and death would surely be beyond the reach of politics.

As I neared the end of my residency at Stanford, fate intervened again with an unexpected offer from Kaiser Permanente. My initial plans to go to South America and provide surgical care for children with cleft lips were suddenly upended by a tragic event—a plastic surgeon at the Kaiser Santa Clara facility had passed away in a plane crash. His colleague reached out to me, seeking temporary help until a permanent replacement could be found. Though I had never set foot in a Kaiser Permanente hospital, I accepted the challenge.

This experience was transformative. I was immediately captivated by the organization's culture and the doctors' unified, mission-driven approach to healthcare. Their dedication to collaborative and supportive practice opened my eyes to the benefits of an integrated healthcare system funded through capitation. This chance occurrence not only altered my career trajectory but also reshaped my entire outlook on medical practice.

My journey took another unexpected turn when I was thrust into a leadership role within The Permanente Medical Group amid an internal crisis. The CEO had suddenly retired, and the organization faced potential bankruptcy. I didn't desire the role, knowing it would limit the time I could spend in surgery. Although reluctant, the unwillingness of other qualified candidates compelled me to accept the challenge. This decision marked the beginning of my second career (after surgeon) and made it possible for me to be where I am today: in this, my third career as author, Stanford professor, keynote speaker, consultant, and podcast host.

Each of these pivotal moments in my life underscores a valuable lesson, taught to me by the words of a longtime mentor: "Windows open and windows close. When a window opens, you better be ready to jump through it." That lesson has never applied more than where American healthcare finds itself today.

For decades, public-health experts and medical professionals have searched for the magic pill, the secret elixir, the silver bullet that would cure the ills of our nation's floundering healthcare system. Professionals across the medical spectrum have sought a breakthrough that could harmonize the disjointed elements of American healthcare, marrying optimal patient care with financial sustainability, and infusing technology with genuine human benefit. In other words, throughout the 21st century, medicine has been looking for a miracle.

In November 2022, ChatGPT emerged as if out of nowhere. There is no evidence that the research pioneers pursued development of a large language model specifically for medicine. And yet, as if by serendipity, we find ourselves with the tool healthcare leaders have needed and sought for decades—a technology capable of simultaneously raising quality, increasing access, and making medical care affordable for all Americans.

How effectively and broadly we apply it will depend on the vision, courage, and efforts of humans. ChatGPT can be used merely as an upgraded search engine for patients and a task-automation tool for doctors. And if those become its primary uses, it will sit on the fringes of the medical system and eventually become yet another example of a powerful technology that was undervalued and underutilized—ultimately failing to benefit patients.

Alternatively, ChatGPT can be used to empower humanity with medical expertise, reduce demand on doctors, and provide patients and physicians alike with the means and ability to reclaim control of healthcare. It can save hundreds of thousands of lives annually and rescue the medical profession from a state of almost universal burnout. But it will only do this if we embrace it. The moment to decide has arrived. The opportunity is now.

***

In a world where change is the only constant, the swift currents of modern life contrast starkly with the sluggish pace of genetic evolution—and of American healthcare, too. Two relatively recent scientific discoveries demonstrate how the very genetic traits that once secured humanity's survival are failing to keep up with the times, producing dire medical consequences. These important biological events offer insights into American medicine—along with a warning about what can happen when humans and healthcare systems fail to change.

For decades, scientists were baffled by what seemed like an evolutionary contradiction.

Sickle cell disease is a condition resulting from a genetic mutation that produces malformed red blood cells. It afflicts approximately one in 365 Black Americans, causing severe pain and organ failure.

Its horrific impact on people raises a question: how has this genetic mutation persisted for 7,300 years? Nature is a merciless editor of life, and so you would expect that across seven millennia, people with this inherited problem would be less likely to survive and reproduce. This curiosity seems to defy the teachings of Charles Darwin, who theorized that evolution discards what no longer serves the survival of a species.

Scientists solved this genetic puzzle in 2011, illuminating a significant evolutionary trade-off.

People living with sickle cell disease have two abnormal genes, one inherited from each parent. While the disease itself affects a large population (roughly 100,000 African Americans), it turns out that a far larger population in the United States carries one "abnormal" gene and one normal gene (comprising as many as 3 million Americans).

This so-called sickle cell trait presents milder symptoms or none at all when compared to the full disease. And, unlike those with the disease, individuals who live with one (but not both) abnormal genes possess a distinct evolutionary advantage: they have a resistance to severe malaria, which every year claims more than 600,000 lives around the globe.

This genetic adaptation (resistance to malaria) kept people alive for many millennia in equatorial Africa, protecting them from the continent's deadliest infectious disease. But in present-day America, malaria is not a major public-health concern due to several factors, including the widespread use of window screens and air conditioning, controlled and limited habitats for the Anopheles mosquitoes (which transmit the disease), and a strong healthcare system capable of managing and containing outbreaks. Therefore, the sickle cell trait is of little value in the United States while sickle cell disease is a cruel, life-threatening problem.

The lesson: genetic changes beneficial in one environment, such as malaria-prone areas, can become harmful in another. This lesson isn't limited to sickle cell disease.

A similar genetic phenomenon was uncovered through research that was published at the start of 2024 in the journal *Nature*. This time, scientists discovered an ancient genetic mutation that is, today, linked to multiple sclerosis.

Their research began with data showing that people living in Northern Europe have twice the number of cases of MS per 100,000 individuals as people in the South of Europe. Like sickle cell disease, MS is a terrible affliction—with immune cells attacking neurons in the brain, interfering with both walking and talking.

Having identified this two-fold variance in the prevalence of MS, scientists compared the genetic makeup of the people in Europe with MS versus those without this devastating problem. And they discovered a correlation between a specific mutated gene and the risk of developing MS. Using archaeological material, the researchers then connected the introduction of this gene into Northern Europe with cattle, goat and sheep herders from Russia who migrated west as far back as 5,000 years ago.

Suddenly, the explanation comes into focus. Thousands of years ago, this genetic abnormality helped protect herders from livestock disease, which at the time was the greatest threat to their survival. However, in the modern era, this same mutation results in an overactive immune response, leading to the development of MS. Once again, a trait that was positive in a specific environmental and historical context has become harmful in today's world.

Just as genetic traits can shift from beneficial to detrimental with changing circumstances, healthcare practices that were once lifesaving can become problematic as medical capabilities advance and societal needs evolve.

Fee-for-service payments, still the most prevalent reimbursement model in American healthcare, reminds us of the need to evolve. In the 1930s, this "mutation" emerged as a solution to the Great Depression. Organizations like Blue Cross began providing health insurance, ensuring healthcare affordability for struggling Americans in need of hospitalization while guaranteeing appropriate compensation for medical providers. FFS, which linked payments to the quantity of care delivered, proved beneficial when the problems physicians treated were acute, one-time issues (e.g., appendicitis, trauma, pneumonia) and relatively inexpensive to resolve. Today, the widespread prevalence of chronic diseases in six out of 10 Americans underlines the limitations of the fee-for-service model. In contrast to "pay for value" models, FFS, with its "pay-for-volume" approach, fails to prioritize preventive services, the avoidance of chronic-disease complications, or the elimination of redundant treatments through coordinated, team-based care. This erodes the excellence of medical care, resulting in higher healthcare costs without corresponding improvements in quality.

This situation is reminiscent of the genetic mutations of sickle cell disease and MS. In contrast to evolution, where biologic change happens solely by chance and takes lifetimes to unfold, humans in medicine can do much better.

Unfortunately, we rarely seize the opportunity. Research demonstrates that it takes 17 years on average for a proven innovation in healthcare to become common practice. When it comes to evolution of healthcare delivery and financing, the pace of change is even more glacial. In 1932, the Committee on the Cost of Medical Care concluded that better clinical outcomes would be achieved if doctors (a) worked in groups rather than as fragmented solo practices and (b) were paid based on the value they provided, rather than just the volume of work they did.

Nearly a century later, these improvements remain elusive. Well-led medical groups remain the minority of all practices in the United States while fee-for-service is still the dominant means by which doctors and hospitals are paid.

Humans have a unique ability to anticipate challenges and proactively implement solutions. Consequently, change in healthcare doesn't have to be random and painfully slow. American medicine, unlike biology, can advance rapidly in response to new knowledge and societal needs. And unlike the DNA in our bodies, humans have the opportunity to consciously adapt to changes in the world around us—leveraging our expertise, technology, and collaborative skills to make it happen.

Standing in the way is a combination of fear (of the risks involved), culture (the norms doctors learn in training) and lack of leadership (the ability to translate vision into action).

The advent of generative AI opens the window for profound change, presenting doctors and patients alike with a chance to build something transformative. The four pillars needed to support the transformation are clear: integration, capitation, cutting-edge technology, and visionary leadership. Along the way, healthcare professionals must encourage patient empowerment, trusting them to take charge of their own health. Regulatory bodies and policymakers will need to update antiquated restrictions, balancing innovation with safeguards against the threats of security breaches, privacy invasions, and the spread of misinformation. As a nation, we will have to abandon the "middlemen mentality" and march forward, boldly, despite the inherent challenges and uncertainties we will encounter.

Serendipity brought ChatGPT to the medical profession. The critical question remains: will we seize this opportunity?

When I asked my coauthor for its concluding thoughts on this question, ChatGPT responded with these wise words: "Serendipity is not just about being at the right place at the right time. It's about recognizing the potential in the unexpected and having the courage to act upon it. It's about seeing beyond the immediate, harnessing the power of insight, and turning chance encounters into pivotal moments that can redefine our path."

Recognition, courage, vision, action: these are the skills that will be necessary.

In closing this exploration of healthcare's future and the role ChatGPT will play, I'm reminded of a poignant moment from my high school days that left me with an unforgettable lesson. An astronaut, one of the pioneers who had ventured into outer space, was invited to share his experiences. After our guest taught us about the US space program and the beauty of the cosmos, a student stepped up to the microphone and asked the man: "What gave you the courage to go into space with all the risks involved?"

With a calm certainty that echoed through the auditorium, the astronaut replied, "When you have the opportunity to do something greater than yourself, you always take it."

For clinicians and patients alike, regaining control of medicine represents such an opportunity. As we stand on the brink of a new era, marked by the promise of generative AI and patient empowerment, we are all astronauts in our own right, embarking on a high-risk mission to redefine the future. It is a venture fraught with challenges, yet rich with the potential for monumental achievements. For every clinician, patient, and participant in this healthcare odyssey, the path forward is not just a professional obligation, but a noble pursuit—a chance to create a legacy that will transcend the individual and preserve the health of generations to come.

ACKNOWLEDGEMENTS

In crafting *ChatGPT, MD*, I have been fortunate to be surrounded and supported by an extraordinary group of individuals and groundbreaking technologies, each contributing uniquely to this journey.

First, the humans who made this book possible:

I owe a debt of gratitude to my longtime friend and writing partner, Ben Lincoln. Ben's story as a patient and his unwavering support have been instrumental in bringing this book to life. He has been a cornerstone of not only this project but also my previous works, "Mistreated" and "Uncaring." His insights, encouragement, and partnership have been invaluable to my work as an author.

Special thanks go to Clayton Smith for his expertise in self-publishing, ensuring this book's successful launch. Jonathan Pliego's exceptional graphic design talents have given *ChatGPT, MD* a visual identity that resonates with its content, and Zach Tarvin's insights into generative AI have enriched my understanding and use of this transformative technology.

In addition, I'm grateful to the 60,000-plus subscribers of my digital newsletters, "Breaking The Rules of Healthcare" (on LinkedIn) and "Monthly Musings on American Healthcare." The readers are active, vocal and passionate; and their votes ultimately decided both the subtitle and cover design for this book.

I appreciate greatly the innovative medical and research efforts of visionary leaders like Dr. Devi Shetty and Dr. Gabriel Escobar, whose success provided inspirational stories for inclusion in *ChatGPT, MD*. I am forever grateful to the patients who trusted me for their medical care both within Kaiser Permanente and on global surgical missions. They fuel my passion for healthcare.

I thank the thousands of clinicians in The Permanente Medical Group, the care-delivery half of Kaiser Permanente, whom I've had the honor of calling colleagues. Their dedication, expertise, and compassion have not only shaped my career but also enriched my understanding of what it means to deliver exceptional care. Their collective commitment to excellence and innovation has been a constant source of inspiration, pushing me to explore new frontiers in healthcare.

Finally, and most important, my heartfelt appreciation belongs to Janet Chao, my fiancée and life-partner. Your support and shared commitment to medicine have been a constant source of joy and inspiration.

Next, a special thanks to the technologies that helped bring this book to life:

ChatGPT, MD would not exist without the incredible capabilities of ChatGPT. Our collaboration has not only expedited the writing process but also opened my eyes to the potential of generative AI in revolutionizing healthcare. The contributions of various AI tools like Gemini, Copilot, and others have been noteworthy, each playing a part in this project's success.

My thanks also extend to the technological tools that facilitated this book's creation, from composition tools like Microsoft Word and Google Docs to Grammarly and PerfectIt for their editing prowess. The analytics from Readable.io and the layout assistance from In-Design have been indispensable. A nod to Midjourney for its role in crafting the book's cover, and a broad thank you to the companies behind these and many other innovations on which I rely—OpenAI, Microsoft, Alphabet, Adobe, Apple, Amazon, and more—for their role in shaping a more connected and efficient world.

This book stands as a testament to what can be achieved when human ingenuity meets technological advancement, and I am deeply thankful to everyone who has been a part of this journey.

BIBLIOGRAPHY

The following bibliography is not intended to be comprehensive. Rather, it is meant as a resource for those who wish to learn more about the technologies powering medicine's future and the context that surrounds American healthcare today. This bibliography includes references to some of my journalistic works, including articles published in Forbes, Harvard Business Review, USA Today, and other outlets. Each offers a deeper perspective on the subject matter included in these pages. For additional information and insight into the chapters of this book, visit RobertPearlMD.com.

Works cited appear in the order of their reference within each chapter.

PART ONE | GENERATIONS

1. The Evolution of Medical Miracles

Cooper, David KC. "Christiaan Barnard—the Surgeon Who Dared: The Story of the First Human-to-Human Heart Transplant." Global Cardiology Science and Practice 2018, no. 2 (July 23, 2018). doi.org/10.21542/gcsp.2018.11.

Hoffenberg, R. "Christiaan Barnard: His First Transplants and Their Impact on Concepts of Death." BMJ 323, no. 7327 (December 22, 2001): 1478–80. doi.org/10.1136/bmj.323.7327.1478.

Silbergleit, Allen. "Norman E. Shumway and the Early Heart Transplants." Texas Heart Institute journal, 2006. ncbi.nlm.nih.gov/pmc/articles/PMC1524691/.

"Norman Shumway, Heart Transplantation Pioneer, Dies at 83." Stanford University News Center, February 10, 2006. med.stanford.edu/news/all-news/2006/02/norman-shumway-heart-transplantation-pioneer-dies-at-83.html.

McKellar, Shelley. "Making a Case for Medical Miracles." Canadian Medical Association Journal 182, no. 6 (March 22, 2010): 595–96. doi.org/10.1503/cmaj.091943.

Duffin, Jacalyn. Medical miracles: Doctors, saints, and healing in the modern world. New York, N.Y. Oxford University Press, 2014.

Stehlik, Josef, Leah B. Edwards, Anna Y. Kucheryavaya, et al. "The Registry of the International Society for Heart and Lung Transplantation: 29th Official Adult Heart Transplant Report—2012." The Journal of Heart and Lung Transplantation 31, no. 10 (October 2012): 1052–64. doi.org/10.1016/j.healun.2012.08.002.

Colvin, M., J.M. Smith, Y. Ahn, M.A. Skeans, et al. "OPTN/SRTR 2019 Annual Data Report: Heart." American Journal of Transplantation 21 (February 2021): 356–440. doi.org/10.1111/ajt.16492.

Abdullahi, Aminu. "Generative AI Models: A Complete Guide." eWEEK, January 9, 2024. eweek.com/artificial-intelligence/generative-ai-model/.

Lawton, George. "Generative Models: Vaes, Gans, Diffusion, Transformers, Nerfs." Enterprise AI, April 19, 2023. techtarget.com/searchenterpriseai/tip/Generative-models-VAEs-GANs-diffusion-transformers-NeRFs.

ChatGPT, November 2022. chat.openai.com.

"Preliminary Estimated Full Year 2019 and December 2019 U.S. Airline Traffic Data." Preliminary Estimated Full Year 2019 and December 2019 U.S. Airline Traffic Data | Bureau of Transportation Statistics. bts.gov/newsroom/preliminary-estimated-full-year-2019-and-december-2019-us-airline-traffic-data.

2. ChatGPT and the Next Frontier

Newman-Toker, David E, Najlla Nassery, et al. "Burden of Serious Harms from Diagnostic Error in the USA." BMJ Quality & Safety 33, no. 2 (July 17, 2023): 109–20. doi.org/10.1136/bmjqs-2021-014130.

Makary, Martin A, and Michael Daniel. "Medical Error—the Third Leading Cause of Death in the US." BMJ, May 3, 2016, i2139. doi.org/10.1136/bmj.i2139.

Porter, Justin, Cynthia Boyd, M. Reza Skandari, and Neda Laiteerapong. "Revisiting the Time Needed to Provide Adult Primary Care." Journal of General Internal Medicine 38, no. 1 (July 1, 2022): 147–55. doi.org/10.1007/s11606-022-07707-x.

Bedayn, Jesse. "States Confront Medical Debt That's Bankrupting Millions." AP News, April 17, 2023. apnews.com/article/medical-debt-legislation-2a4f2fab7e2c58a68ac4541b8309c7aa.

Tai-Seale, Ming, Thomas G. McGuire, and Weimin Zhang. "Time Allocation in Primary Care Office Visits." Health Services Research 42, no. 5 (January 24, 2007): 1871–94. doi.org/10.1111/j.1475-6773.2006.00689.x.

Reed, Tina. "The Doctor Will Fee You Now." Axios, February 6, 2024. axios.com/2024/02/26/doctor-appointment-fees-costs.

Sinsky, Christine A., Roger L. Brown, Martin J. Stillman, and Mark Linzer. "Covid-Related Stress and Work Intentions in a Sample of US Health Care Workers." Mayo Clinic Proceedings: Innovations, Quality & Outcomes 5, no. 6 (December 2021): 1165–73. doi.org/10.1016/j.mayocpiqo.2021.08.007.

Shanafelt, Tait D., Liselotte N. Dyrbye, et al. "Career Plans of US Physicians after the First 2 Years of the COVID-19 Pandemic." Mayo Clinic Proceedings 98, no. 11 (November 2023): 1629–40. doi.org/10.1016/j.mayocp.2023.07.006.

Van Alstin, Chad. "Apple Vision Pro App Brings Augmented Reality to Radiology." Health Imaging, February 7, 2024. healthimaging.com/topics/health-it/enterprise-imaging/visage-ease-apple-vision-pro-virtual-augmented-reality-radiology.

Regina Ta, Nicol Turner Lee, Niam Yaraghi, et al. "Generative AI in Health Care: Opportunities, Challenges, and Policy." Brookings, January 31, 2024. brookings.edu/articles/generative-ai-in-health-care-opportunities-challenges-and-policy/.

Chen, Yan, and Pouyan Esmaeilzadeh. "Generative AI in Medical Practice: In-Depth Exploration of Privacy and Security Challenges." Journal of Medical Internet Research 26 (March 8, 2024). doi.org/10.2196/53008.

Tyson, Alec. "60% of Americans Would Be Uncomfortable with Provider Relying on AI in Their Own Health Care." Pew Research Center Science & Society, February 22, 2023. pewresearch.org/science/2023/02/22/60-of-americans-would-be-uncomfortable-with-provider-relying-on-ai-in-their-own-health-care/.

Loeb, Eric. "Bot Docs? Not Likely: 69% of US Adults Uncomfortable Being Diagnosed by Ai." Salesforce, March 7, 2024. salesforce.com/news/stories/ai-in-healthcare-research/.

"Leading Strategic Change in the Health Care Industry (STRAMGT 581)." Stanford University Graduate School of Business course catalog, 2023. explorecourses.stanford.edu/.

"The Five Forces." The Five Forces - Institute For Strategy And Competitiveness - Harvard Business School. Accessed March 20, 2024. isc.hbs.edu/strategy/business-strategy/Pages/the-five-forces.aspx.

Pearl, Robert. "Amazon, CVS, Walmart Are Playing Healthcare's Long Game." Forbes, October 12, 2022. forbes.com/sites/robertpearl/2022/10/10/amazon-cvs-walmart-are-playing-healthcares-long-game/.

Pearl, Robert. Mistreated: Why we think we're getting good health care and why we're usually wrong. New York: PublicAffairs, 2017.

Pearl, Robert. Uncaring: How the culture of medicine kills doctors and patients. New York: PublicAffairs, 2021.

Hu, Krystal. "ChatGPT Sets Record for Fastest-Growing User Base." Reuters, February 2, 2023. reuters.com/technology/chatgpt-sets-record-fastest-growing-user-base-analyst-note-2023-02-01/.

Metz, Cade. "Chatbots May 'hallucinate' More Often than Many Realize." The New York Times, November 6, 2023. nytimes.com/2023/11/06/technology/chatbots-hallucination-rates.html.

3. The Life and Times of American Medicine

Willis, Charles A. "Destination America: When Did They Come?" PBS. Accessed March 20, 2024. pbs.org/destinationamerica/usim_wn_noflash_6.html.

Bibliography

"Pogroms." United States holocaust memorial museum: Holocaust Encyclopedia. Accessed March 20, 2024. encyclopedia.ushmm.org/content/en/article/pogroms.

Chovatiya, Raj, and Jonathan I. Silverberg. "Inpatient Morbidity and Mortality of Measles in the United States." PLOS ONE 15, no. 4 (April 28, 2020). doi.org/10.1371/journal.pone.0231329.

Dalen, James E., Joseph S. Alpert, Robert J. Goldberg, and Ronald S. Weinstein. "The Epidemic of the 20th Century: Coronary Heart Disease." The American Journal of Medicine 127, no. 9 (September 2014): 807–12. doi.org/10.1016/j.amjmed.2014.04.015.

Fornasieri, Valerie W., and Abraham Verghese. "Reviews and Notes: Textbook of Physical Diagnosis: History and Examination; and Physical Diagnosis: Bedside Evaluation of Diagnosis and Function." Annals of Internal Medicine 122, no. 12 (June 15, 1995): 965. doi.org/10.7326/0003-4819-122-12-199506150-00028.

Meyer, Harriet S., David H. Morse, and Robert Hogan. "20th Century Medicine." JAMA 285, no. 21 (June 6, 2001): 2790. doi.org/10.1001/jama.285.21.2790-jbk0606-6-1.

4. Healthcare's Unfulfilled Promises

Van De Belt, Tom H, Lucien JLPG Engelen, et al. "Definition of Health 2.0 and Medicine 2.0: A Systematic Review." Journal of Medical Internet Research 12, no. 2 (June 11, 2010). doi.org/10.2196/jmir.1350.

Sanders, Dale. "Healthcare 2.0: The Age of Analytics." Health Catalyst. Lecture, 2013.

ZDoggMD. "The Health 3.0 Movement." ZDoggMD, July 6, 2021. zdoggmd.com/health-3-point-0/.

Nash, David B. "Health 3.0." P & T : a peer-reviewed journal for formulary management, February 2008. ncbi.nlm.nih.gov/pmc/articles/PMC2730068/.

Chen, Chiehfeng, El-Wui Loh, Ken N. Kuo, and Ka-Wai Tam. "The Times They Are A-Changin' – Healthcare 4.0 Is Coming!" Journal of Medical Systems 44, no. 2 (December 23, 2019). doi.org/10.1007/s10916-019-1513-0.

deBronkart, Dave. "From Patient Centered to People Powered: Autonomy on the Rise." BMJ, February 10, 2015. doi.org/10.1136/bmj.h148.

Yap, Janson, and Yong Chern Chet. "Healthcare 3.0." Healthcare 3.0: Healthcare for the new normal, 2013. www2.deloitte.com/content/dam/Deloitte/sg/Documents/life-sciences-health-care/sg-lshc-healthcare-3.0-no-exp.pdf.

Li, Jingshan, and Pascale Carayon. "Health Care 4.0: A Vision for Smart and Connected Health Care." IISE Transactions on Healthcare Systems Engineering, February 15, 2021, 1–10. doi.org/10.1080/24725579.2021.1884627.

Mearian, Lucas. "The Fax Is Still King in Healthcare - and It's Not Going Away Anytime Soon." Computerworld, May 22, 2023. computerworld.com/article/3697270/the-fax-is-still-king-in-healthcare-and-its-not-going-away-anytime-soon.html.

Panner, Morris. "The CD-ROM's Last Holdout: Your Doctor's Office." Forbes, August 1, 2022. forbes.com/sites/forbestechcouncil/2022/07/28/the-cd-roms-last-holdout-your-doctors-office/.

Pearl, Robert, and Brian Wayling. "The Telehealth Era Is Just Beginning." Harvard Business Review no. May-June, 2022.

Gorn, David. "These Doctors Think Electronic Health Records Are Hurting Their Relationships with Patients." PBS News Hour, July 21, 2017. pbs.org/newshour/health/doctors-think-electronic-health-records-hurting-relationships-patients.

Howard, Ryan. "How Collaboration Can Drastically Improve U.S. Health Care." Harvard Business Review, March 16, 2022. hbr.org/2022/03/how-collaboration-can-drastically-improve-u-s-health-care.

Pratt, Rebekah, Beth Gyllstrom, Kim Gearin, et al. "Identifying Barriers to Collaboration between Primary Care and Public Health: Experiences at the Local Level." Public Health Reports 133, no. 3 (April 3, 2018): 311–17. doi.org/10.1177/0033354918764391.

Li, Edmond, Jonathan Clarke, Hutan Ashrafian, Ara Darzi, and Ana Luisa Neves. "The Impact of Electronic Health Record Interoperability on Safety and Quality of Care in High-Income Countries: Systematic Review." Journal of Medical Internet Research 24, no. 9 (September 15, 2022). doi.org/10.2196/38144.

Pearl, Robert. "The Mystery of the Hospital Industry's Silence over EHR Rule Proposal." Forbes, March 9, 2020. forbes.com/sites/robertpearl/2020/03/08/the-curious-case-ehr-rule/.

Pearl, Robert. "Hard Cases: The Multibillion-Dollar Bet on Health It." LinkedIn, March 8, 2018. linkedin.com/pulse/hard-cases-multibillion-dollar-bet-health-robert-pearl-m-d-/.

Pearl, Robert. "Managing the Most Expensive Patients." Harvard Business Review, February 26, 2020. hbr.org/2020/01/managing-the-most-expensive-patients.

"Q&A: Dr. Robert Pearl's Take on Challenges with Integrated Delivery …" Modern Healthcare, 2017. modernhealthcare.com/article/20161231/MAGAZINE/312319957/q-a-dr-robert-pearl-s-take-on-challenges-with-integrated-delivery-systems.

Levin, Theodore R., Douglas A. Corley, et al. "Effects of Organized Colorectal Cancer Screening on Cancer Incidence and Mortality in a Large Community-Based Population." Gastroenterology 155, no. 5 (November 2018). doi.org/10.1053/j.gastro.2018.07.017.

Sidney, Stephen, Michael E. Sorel, Charles P. Quesenberry, et al. "Comparative Trends in Heart Disease, Stroke, and All-Cause Mortality in the United States and a Large Integrated Healthcare Delivery System." The American Journal of Medicine 131, no. 7 (July 2018). doi.org/10.1016/j.amjmed.2018.02.014.

"American Heart Association Recognizes Kaiser Permanente Northern California Hospitals for Commitment to Reducing Death and Disability among Cardiac and Stroke Patients." Kaiser Permanente Look insideKP Northern California, July 18, 2023. nlookinside.kaiserpermanente.org/american-heart-association-recognizes-kaiser-permanente-northern-california-hospitals-for-commitment-to-reducing-death-and-disability-among-cardiac-and-stroke-patients/.

Lesser, Cara S., Paul B. Ginsburg, and Kelly J. Devers. "The End of an Era: What Became of the 'Managed Care Revolution' in 2001?" Health Services Research 38, no. 1p2 (February 2003): 337–55. doi.org/10.1111/1475-6773.00119.

Mechanic, David. "The Rise and Fall of Managed Care." Journal of Health and Social Behavior 45 (2004): 76–86. jstor.org/stable/3653825.

Armour, Stephanie. "Health insurers must streamline prior authorization decisions, new rule says." wsj.com/health/healthcare/u-s-issues-rule-to-speed-up-health-insurers-medical-paperwork-decisions-59ae98fb.

Berg, Sara. "What Doctors Wish Patients Knew about Prior Authorization." American Medical Association, September 11, 2023. ama-assn.org/practice-management/prior-authorization/what-doctors-wish-patients-knew-about-prior-authorization.

"Telehealth Policy Changes after the COVID-19 Public Health Emergency." telehealth.hhs.gov. Accessed March 21, 2024. telehealth.hhs.gov/providers/telehealth-policy/policy-changes-after-the-covid-19-public-health-emergency.

Pearl, Robert. "ChatGPT Will Reduce Clinician Burnout, If Doctors Embrace It." Forbes, December 7, 2023. forbes.com/sites/robertpearl/2023/12/06/chatgpt-will-reduce-clinician-burnout-if-doctors-embrace-it/.

5. Knowledge is Power

Keen, Andrew. "Keen on: A Gutenberg Moment in the History of Medicine: Dr Robert Pearl Offers 5 Ways That Generative AI Is about to Revolutionize Healthcare on Apple Podcasts." Apple Podcasts, March 24, 2023. podcasts.apple.com/us/podcast/a-gutenberg-moment-in-the-history-of-medicine/id1448694012?i=1000605759520.

"Printing Press." Encyclopedia Britannica, March 8, 2024. britannica.com/technology/printing-press.

M, Zul. "How Johannes Gutenberg Transformed the Publishing Industry." PublishingState.com, December 2, 2023. publishingstate.com/how-johannes-gutenberg-transformed-the-publishing-industry/2023/.

Bibliography

Kulikowski, Casimir A. "Beginnings of Artificial Intelligence in Medicine (AIM): Computational Artifice Assisting Scientific Inquiry and Clinical Art – with Reflections on Present AIM Challenges." Yearbook of Medical Informatics 28, no. 01 (April 25, 2019): 249–56. doi.org/10.1055/s-0039-1677895.

Jobs, Steve. "Steve Jobs Introduces iPhone in 2007 at Macworld San Francisco 2007 Keynote Address ." YouTube, October 8, 2011. youtube.com/watch?v=MnrJzXM7a6o.

Isaacson, Walter. "The Real Leadership Lessons of Steve Jobs." Harvard Business Review, October 29, 2014. hbr.org/2012/04/the-real-leadership-lessons-of-steve-jobs.

Hesse, Bradford W. "The Patient, the Physician, and Dr. Google." AMA Journal of Ethics 14, no. 5 (May 1, 2012): 398–402. doi.org/10.1001/virtualmentor.2012.14.5.stas1-1205.

Van Riel, Noor, Koen Auwerx, Pieterjan Debbaut, et al. "The Effect of Dr Google on Doctor–Patient Encounters in Primary Care: A Quantitative, Observational, Cross-Sectional Study." BJGP Open 1, no. 2 (May 16, 2017). doi.org/10.3399/bjgpopen17x100833.

Nimmon, Laura, and Terese Stenfors-Hayes. "The 'Handling' of Power in the Physician-Patient Encounter: Perceptions from Experienced Physicians." BMC Medical Education 16, no. 1 (April 18, 2016). doi.org/10.1186/s12909-016-0634-0.

Kelly, Kevin. "What Ai-Generated Art Really Means for Human Creativity." WIRED, November 17, 2022. wired.com/story/picture-limitless-creativity-ai-image-generators/.

Shanfeld, Ethan. "Ghostwriter's 'heart on My Sleeve,' the AI-Generated Song Mimicking Drake and the Weeknd, Submitted for Grammys." Variety, September 6, 2023. variety.com/2023/music/news/ai-generated-drake-the-weeknd-song-submitted-for-grammys-1235714805/.

"Will AI Render Programming Obsolete?" The MIT Press Reader, January 13, 2024. thereader.mitpress.mit.edu/will-ai-render-programming-obsolete/.

6. The AI Revolution: In ChatGPT's Own Words

ChatGPT, 2024. chat.openai.com/.

"John McCarthy Obituary." The Guardian, October 25, 2011. theguardian.com/technology/2011/oct/25/john-mccarthy.

"Artificial Intelligence (AI) Coined at Dartmouth." Dartmouth. Accessed March 22, 2024. home.dartmouth.edu/about/artificial-intelligence-ai-coined-dartmouth.

Davis, Randall, and Jonathan J. King. "The origin of rule-based systems in AI." Rule-based expert systems: The MYCIN experiments of the Stanford Heuristic Programming Project (1984).

Alowais, Shuroug A., Sahar S. Alghamdi, et al. "Revolutionizing Healthcare: The Role of Artificial Intelligence in Clinical Practice." BMC Medical Education 23, no. 1 (September 22, 2023). doi.org/10.1186/s12909-023-04698-z.

Elkus, Adam. "MYCIN, Watson, and AI History." CTOvision.com, July 20, 2019. ctovision.com/watson-mycin-ai-history/.

Dickson, Ben. "What Is Artificial Narrow Intelligence (Narrow AI)?" TechTalks, April 12, 2020. bdtechtalks.com/2020/04/09/what-is-narrow-artificial-intelligence-ani/.

Yao, Deborah. "25 Years Ago Today: How Deep Blue vs. Kasparov Changed Ai Forever: Ai Business." AI Business Informs, educates and connects the global AI community, November 29, 2023. aibusiness.com/ml/25-years-ago-today-how-deep-blue-vs-kasparov-changed-ai-forever.

Shahid, Nida, Tim Rappon, and Whitney Berta. "Applications of Artificial Neural Networks in Health Care Organizational Decision-Making: A Scoping Review." PLOS ONE 14, no. 2 (February 19, 2019). doi.org/10.1371/journal.pone.0212356.

Zheng, Dan, Xiujing He, and Jing Jing. "Overview of Artificial Intelligence in Breast Cancer Medical Imaging." Journal of Clinical Medicine 12, no. 2 (January 4, 2023): 419. doi.org/10.3390/jcm12020419.

Ahn, Jong Seok, Sangwon Shin, Su-A Yang, Eun Kyung Park, Ki Hwan Kim, Soo Ick Cho, Chan-Young Ock, and Seokhwi Kim. "Artificial Intelligence in Breast Cancer Diagnosis and Personalized Medicine." Journal of Breast Cancer 26, no. 5 (2023): 405. doi.org/10.4048/jbc.2023.26.e45.

DePeau-Wilson, Michael. "Google AI Performs at 'expert' Level on U.S. Medical Licensing Exam." Medical News, March 14, 2023. medpagetoday.com/special-reports/exclusives/103522.

Ayers, John W., Adam Poliak, Mark Dredze, et al. "Comparing Physician and Artificial Intelligence Chatbot Responses to Patient Questions Posted to a Public Social Media Forum." JAMA Internal Medicine 183, no. 6 (June 1, 2023): 589. doi.org/10.1001/jamainternmed.2023.1838.

Pearl, Robert. "More Empathetic: Doctors or CHATGPT?" LinkedIn, August 7, 2023. linkedin.com/pulse/more-empathetic-doctors-chatgpt-robert-pearl-m-d-/.

PART TWO | GENERATIVITY

7. Welcome to Healthcare 4.0

Burda, David. "Podcast: Calculating the ROI of VBC 10/19/23." 4sight Health, October 19, 2023. 4sighthealth.com/podcast-calculating-the-roi-of-vbc-10-19-23/.

Burda, David. "4sight Health Roundup Podcast Transcript ." 4sight Health, October 19, 2023. 4sighthealth.com/wp-content/uploads/2023/10/4sight-Health-Roundup-podcast-transcript-10-19-23.pdf.

Visan, Anita Ioana, and Irina Negut. "Integrating Artificial Intelligence for Drug Discovery in the Context of Revolutionizing Drug Delivery." Life 14, no. 2 (February 7, 2024): 233. doi.org/10.3390/life14020233.

"Global Trends in R&D 2024: Activity, Productivity, and Enablers." IQVIA, 2024. iqvia.com/insights/the-iqvia-institute/reports-and-publications/reports/global-trends-in-r-and-d-2024-activity-productivity-and-enablers.

Reddy, Sandeep. "Generative AI in Healthcare: An Implementation Science Informed Translational Path on Application, Integration and Governance." Implementation Science 19, no. 1 (March 15, 2024). doi.org/10.1186/s13012-024-01357-9.

Pearl, Robert. "5 Ways ChatGPT Will Change Healthcare Forever, for Better." Forbes, October 5, 2023. forbes.com/sites/robertpearl/2023/02/13/5-ways-chatgpt-will-change-healthcare-forever-for-better/.

DePeau-Wilson, Michael. "GPT-4 Is Here. How Can Doctors Use Generative AI Now?" Medical News, March 20, 2023. medpagetoday.com/special-reports/exclusives/103616.

Hashimoto, Daniel A, Guy Rosman, Daniela Rus, and Ozanan R Meireles. "Artificial Intelligence in Surgery: Promises and Perils." Annals of surgery, July 2018. ncbi.nlm.nih.gov/pmc/articles/PMC5995666/.

"How Generative AI Has Revolutionized Robotic Surgery." AiiotTalk, November 18, 2023. aiiottalk.com/generative-ai-has-revolutionized-robotic-surgery/.

Vuksanaj, Kathy. "Generative AI and Precision Medicine--the Future Is Not What It Used to Be." Inside Precision Medicine, November 21, 2023. insideprecisionmedicine.com/news-and-features/generative-ai-and-precision-medicine-the-future-is-not-what-it-used-to-be/.

Johnson, Khari. "ChatGPT Can Help Doctors-and Hurt Patients." Wired, April 24, 2023. wired.com/story/chatgpt-can-help-doctors-and-hurt-patients/.

"AAMC Report Reinforces Mounting Physician Shortage." AAMC, June 11, 2021. aamc.org/news/press-releases/aamc-report-reinforces-mounting-physician-shortage.

Porter, Justin, Cynthia Boyd, M. Reza Skandari, and Neda Laiteerapong. "Revisiting the Time Needed to Provide Adult Primary Care." Journal of General Internal Medicine 38, no. 1 (July 1, 2022): 147–55. doi.org/10.1007/s11606-022-07707-x.

Kharraz, Oliver. "Long Waits to See a Doctor Are a Public Health Crisis." STAT, May 1, 2023. statnews.com/2023/05/02/doctor-appointment-wait-times-solutions/.

Pearl, Robert. "Transforming Primary Care by Breaking the Rules." Robert Pearl, MD, December 5, 2023. robertpearlmd.com/breaking-the-rules/.

Pearl, Robert. "Healthcare Leadership: Following the Money Can Lead to Positive Change." Forbes, December 1, 2022. forbes.com/sites/robertpearl/2022/11/29/healthcare-leadership-following-the-money-can-lead-to-positive-change/.

Pearl, Robert. "Robert Pearl: Fee-for-Service Model Hampers American Health Care System, the Worst among Wealthy Nations." Rochester Post Bulletin, October 23, 2021. postbulletin.com/opinion/columns/robert-pearl-fee-for-service-model-hampers-american-health-care-system-the-worst-among-wealthy-nations.

8. A First Look at AI Empowerment

Bhasker, Shashank, Damien Bruce, Jessica Lamb, and George Stein. "Generative AI in Healthcare: The End of Administrative Burdens for Workers." C3 AI, January 11, 2024. c3.ai/generative-ai-in-healthcare-the-end-of-administrative-burdens-for-workers/.

Matias, Yossi. "Our Progress on Generative AI in Health." Google, March 19, 2024. blog.google/technology/health/google-generative-ai-healthcare/.

MacMillan, Carrie. "Generative AI for Health Information: A Guide to Safe Use." Yale Medicine, January 8, 2024. yalemedicine.org/news/generative-ai-artificial-intelligence-for-health-info.

Natalie Schibell, MPH. "Generative AI's Role in Elevating Patient Care and Self-Management." Physicians Practice, March 22, 2024. physicianspractice.com/view/generative-ai-s-role-in-elevating-patient-care-and-self-management.

Reddy, Sandeep. "Generative AI in Healthcare: An Implementation Science Informed Translational Path on Application, Integration and Governance - Implementation Science." BioMed Central, March 15, 2024. implementationscience.biomedcentral.com/articles/10.1186/s13012-024-01357-9.

Berger, Eric, KC George, Nirad Jain, et al. "Generative AI Will Transform Healthcare." Bain, March 20, 2024. bain.com/insights/generative-ai-global-healthcare-private-equity-report-2024/.

"Generative AI to Reshape the Future of Health Care." Deloitte United States, November 22, 2023. www2.deloitte.com/us/en/pages/life-sciences-and-health-care/articles/generative-ai-in-healthcare.html.

"AI in Remote Patient Monitoring: The Top 4 Use Cases in 2024." HealthSnap, Inc., March 11, 2024. healthsnap.io/ai-in-remote-patient-monitoring-the-top-4-use-cases-in-2024/.

Filbin, Patrick. "How Generative AI Is Being Used in Home-Based Care." Home Health Care News, August 8, 2023. homehealthcarenews.com/2023/08/how-generative-ai-is-being-used-in-home-based-care/.

"Why Generative AI in Healthcare Requires a Focus on Caregivers and Patients: Healthcare IT Today." Healthcare IT Today, October 16, 2023. healthcareittoday.com/2023/10/17/why-generative-ai-in-healthcare-requires-a-focus-on-caregivers-and-patients/.

Giansanti, Daniele. "The Artificial Intelligence in Teledermatology: A Narrative Review on Opportunities, Perspectives, and Bottlenecks." International Journal of Environmental Research and Public Health 20, no. 10 (May 12, 2023): 5810. doi.org/10.3390/ijerph20105810.

Ravindran, Sandeep. "Here Come the Artificial Intelligence Nutritionists." The New York Times, March 14, 2022. nytimes.com/2022/03/14/well/eat/ai-diet-personalized.html.

Galmarini, Carlos María. "Nutritional Ai: Making Our Shopping Baskets Healthier." OpenMind, February 2, 2024. bbvaopenmind.com/en/science/research/nutritional-ai-making-our-shopping-baskets-healthier/.

"Can an AI-Powered Fitness App Outperform a Human Trainer?" CNET. Accessed March 22, 2024. cnet.com/tech/can-an-ai-powered-fitness-app-outperform-a-human-trainer/.

Clark, Michelle, and Melissa Severn. "Artificial Intelligence in Prehospital Emergency Health Care." National Center for Biotechnology Information. June 15, 2023. ncbi.nlm.nih.gov/books/NBK596747/.

Ganjavi, Conner, Michael B Eppler, Asli Pekcan, et al. "Publishers' and Journals' Instructions to Authors on Use of Generative Artificial Intelligence in Academic and Scientific Publishing: Bibliometric Analysis." BMJ, January 31, 2024. doi.org/10.1136/bmj-2023-077192.

Pearl, Robert. "3 Ways ChatGPT's 'Memory' Can Spark Breakthroughs in Healthcare." Forbes, March 21, 2024. forbes.com/sites/robertpearl/2024/03/18/why-chatgpts-memory-will-be-a-healthcare-gamechanger/.

Pearl, Robert. "The AI-Empowered Patient Is Coming: Are Doctors Ready?" Forbes, October 6, 2023. forbes.com/sites/robertpearl/2023/10/04/the-ai-empowered-patient-is-coming-are-doctors-ready/.

9. Fixing Medicine's Biggest Problems

"Chronic Diseases in America." Centers for Disease Control and Prevention, December 13, 2022. cdc.gov/chronicdisease/resources/infographic/chronic-diseases.htm.

"Health and Economic Benefits of Diabetes Interventions." Centers for Disease Control and Prevention, December 21, 2022. cdc.gov/chronicdisease/programs-impact/pop/diabetes.htm.

McCarthy, Douglas, Kimberly Mueller, and Jennifer Wrenn. "Kaiser Permanente Case Study." The Commonwealth Fund, 2009. commonwealthfund.org/sites/default/files/documents/___media_files_publications_case_study_2009_jun_1278_mccarthy_kaiser_case_study_624_update.pdf.

Jaffe, Marc G., and Joseph D. Young. "The Kaiser Permanente Northern California Story: Improving Hypertension Control from 44% to 90% in 13 Years (2000 to 2013)." The Journal of Clinical Hypertension 18, no. 4 (March 3, 2016): 260–61. doi.org/10.1111/jch.12803.

Rosenthal, Elisabeth. "The Shrinking Number of Primary Care Physicians Is Reaching a Tipping Point." KFF Health News, September 8, 2023. kffhealthnews.org/news/article/lack-of-primary-care-tipping-point/.

State of the Primary Care Workforce 2023, November 2023. bhw.hrsa.gov/sites/default/files/bureau-health-workforce/data-research/state-of-primary-care-workforce-2023.pdf.

Hassanein, Nada. "A Third of Americans Don't Have a Primary Care Provider, Report Finds." USA Today, February 28, 2023. usatoday.com/story/news/health/2023/02/28/americans-lack-primary-care-provider-report/11359096002/.

"Financing: The United States Is Underinvesting in Primary Care." Milbank Memorial Fund, March 14, 2023. milbank.org/publications/health-of-us-primary-care-a-baseline-scorecard/i-financing-the-united-states-is-underinvesting-in-primary-care/.

Vogel, Lauren. "Life Expectancy Grows with Supply of Primary Care Doctors." Canadian Medical Association Journal 191, no. 12 (March 24, 2019). doi.org/10.1503/cmaj.109-5729.

"More Primary Care Physicians Leads to Longer Life Spans." News Center, February 18, 2019. med.stanford.edu/news/all-news/2019/02/more-primary-care-physicians-lead-to-longer-life-spans.html.

"Burnout Threatens Primary Care Workforce and Doctors' Mental Health." CBS News, 2023. cbsnews.com/news/doctor-burnout-primary-care-medical-workforce-mental-health/.

"Stressed out and Burned out: The Global Primary Care Crisis." Commonwealth Fund, November 17, 2022. commonwealthfund.org/publications/issue-briefs/2022/nov/stressed-out-burned-out-2022-international-survey-primary-care-physicians.

Pearl, Robert. "Clinician Burnout in the US: New Data, Surprising Insights." LinkedIn, November 28, 2023. linkedin.com/pulse/clinician-burnout-us-new-data-surprising-insights-robert-pearl-m-d--zjenc/.

Pearl, Robert. "ChatGPT Will Reduce Clinician Burnout, If Doctors Embrace It." Forbes, December 7, 2023. forbes.com/sites/robertpearl/2023/12/06/chatgpt-will-reduce-clinician-burnout-if-doctors-embrace-it/.

"High U.S. Health Care Spending: Where Is It All Going?" High U.S. Health Care Spending | Commonwealth Fund, October 4, 2023. commonwealthfund.org/publications/issue-briefs/2023/oct/high-us-health-care-spending-where-is-it-all-going.

Frakt, Austin. "The Astonishingly High Administrative Costs of U.S. Health Care." The New York Times, July 16, 2018. nytimes.com/2018/07/16/upshot/costs-health-care-us.html.

Siwicki, Bill. "How Generative AI Can Help Address the Critical Nursing Shortage." Healthcare IT News, February 16, 2024. healthcareitnews.com/news/how-generative-ai-can-help-address-critical-nursing-shortage.

Eastabrook, Diane. Home Healthcare turns to AI to fill staffing gaps, October 17, 2023. modernhealthcare.com/providers/home-healthcare-ai-staffing-gaps-hospice-hospital-at-home.

Bruce, Giles. "How Mayo, Mass General Brigham, Providence Are Using Generative AI, Virtual Nursing." Becker's Hospital Review, 2023. beckershospitalreview.com/innovation/how-mayo-mass-general-brigham-providence-are-using-generative-ai-virtual-nursing.html.

Chenais, Gabrielle, Emmanuel Lagarde, and Cédric Gil-Jardiné. "Artificial Intelligence in Emergency Medicine: Viewpoint of Current Applications and Foreseeable Opportunities and Challenges." Journal of Medical Internet Research 25 (May 23, 2023). doi.org/10.2196/40031.

JSTEP, Columbia. "Harnessing the Power of AI in Emergency Triage: A Paradigm Shift." Medium, October 25, 2023. medium.com/columbia-journal-of-science-tech-ethics-and-policy/harnessing-the-power-of-ai-in-emergency-triage-a-paradigm-shift-0af7786948bd.

Newman-Toker, David E, Najlla Nassery, et al. "Burden of Serious Harms from Diagnostic Error in the USA." BMJ Quality & Safety 33, no. 2 (July 17, 2023): 109–20. doi.org/10.1136/bmjqs-2021-014130.

Kahneman, Daniel. Thinking fast and slow. U.K. Penguin Books, 2011.

Pearl, Robert. "The Silent Epidemic: How Cognitive Biases Impact Healthcare Decisions." Forbes, January 31, 2024. forbes.com/sites/robertpearl/2024/01/31/the-silent-epidemic-how-cognitive-biases-impact-healthcare-decisions/.

Auerbach, Andrew D., Tiffany M. Lee, et al. "Diagnostic Errors in Hospitalized Adults Who Died or Were Transferred to Intensive Care." JAMA Internal Medicine 184, no. 2 (February 1, 2024): 164. doi.org/10.1001/jamainternmed.2023.7347.

James, John T. "A New, Evidence-Based Estimate of Patient Harms Associated with Hospital Care." Journal of Patient Safety 9, no. 3 (September 2013): 122–28. doi.org/10.1097/pts.0b013e3182948a69.

Zheng, Yifan, Brigid Rowell, Qiyuan Chen, et al. "Designing Human-Centered AI to Prevent Medication Dispensing Errors: Focus Group Study with Pharmacists." JMIR Formative Research 7 (December 25, 2023). doi.org/10.2196/51921.

Kohn, Linda T., Janet M. Corrigan, and Molla S. Donaldson. "To Err Is Human." Institute of Medicine (US) Committee on Quality of Health Care in America, March 1, 2000. doi.org/10.17226/9728.

10. The Doctor-Patient-AI Partnership

"Evescape." EVEscape. Accessed March 22, 2024. evescape.org/.

Caruso, Catherine. "An AI Tool That Can Help Forecast Viral Variants." Harvard Medical School, October 11, 2023. hms.harvard.edu/news/ai-tool-can-help-forecast-viral-outbreaks.

Berg, Sara. "What Doctors Wish Patients Knew about Prior Authorization." American Medical Association, September 11, 2023. ama-assn.org/practice-management/prior-authorization/what-doctors-wish-patients-knew-about-prior-authorization.

Arndt, Brian G., John W. Beasley, Michelle D. Watkinson, et al. "Tethered to the EHR: Primary Care Physician Workload Assessment Using EHR Event Log Data and Time-Motion Observations." The Annals of Family Medicine 15, no. 5 (September 2017): 419–26. doi.org/10.1370/afm.2121.

Tseng, Phillip, Robert S. Kaplan, et al. "Administrative Costs Associated with Physician Billing and Insurance-Related Activities at an Academic Health Care System." JAMA 319, no. 7 (February 20, 2018): 691. doi.org/10.1001/jama.2017.19148.

Pearl, Robert. "How Generative AI Will Upend the Doctor-Patient Relationship." Forbes, October 19, 2023. forbes.com/sites/robertpearl/2023/10/18/how-generative-ai-will-upend-the-doctor-patient-relationship/.

Afzal. "The Flipped Classroom: How Khan Academy Enables a New Model of Learning." Tech in Teach, October 30, 2023. techinteach.com/the-flipped-classroom-how-khan-academy-enables-a-new-model-of-learning/.

Atreja A, Bellam N, Levy SR. Strategies to enhance patient adherence: making it simple. MedGenMed. 2005 Mar 16;7(1):4. PMID: 16369309; PMCID: PMC1681370.

Noer, Michael. "One Man, One Computer, 10 Million Students: How Khan Academy Is Reinventing Education." Forbes, May 15, 2015. forbes.com/sites/michaelnoer/2012/11/02/one-man-one-computer-10-million-students-how-khan-academy-is-reinventing-education/.

PART THREE | GENESIS

11. The Road to AI-Empowered Healthcare

Salvucci, Jeremy. "What Was the Dot-Com Bubble & Why Did It Burst?" The Street, May 31, 2022. thestreet.com/dictionary/dot-com-bubble-and-burst.

Chang, David. "The Subprime Mortgage Crisis of 2008." The Motley Fool, October 26, 2023. fool.com/the-ascent/mortgages/subprime-mortgage-crisis/.

Pifer, Rebecca. "US Health Spending to Surpass $7T by 2031, CMS Actuaries Say." Healthcare Dive, June 15, 2023. healthcaredive.com/news/us-health-spending-projections-cms-covid-ira/652973/.

"Mirror, Mirror: Comparing Health Systems across Countries." Commonwealth Fund, 2021. commonwealthfund.org/series/mirror-mirror-comparing-health-systems-across-countries.

"Historical National Health Expenditures." CMS.gov, 2023. cms.gov/data-research/statistics-trends-and-reports/national-health-expenditure-data/historical.

"U.S. Health Care from a Global Perspective, 2022: Accelerating Spending, Worsening Outcomes." Commonwealth Fund, January 31, 2023. commonwealthfund.org/publications/issue-briefs/2023/jan/us-health-care-global-perspective-2022.

Pearl, Robert. Mistreated: Why we think we're getting good health care and why we're usually wrong. New York: PublicAffairs, 2017.

Pearl, Robert. Uncaring: How the culture of medicine kills doctors and patients. S.l.: PublicAffairs, 2024.

Pearl, Robert. "How America Skimps on Healthcare." Forbes, November 9, 2023. forbes.com/sites/robertpearl/2023/11/08/how-america-skimps-on-healthcare/.

Glatter, Robert D. "Shrinkflation: Less Bang for Your Health Insurance Buck." Medscape, January 11, 2024. medscape.com/viewarticle/999167.

McGough, Matthew, Matthew McGough, et al. "How Has U.S. Spending on Healthcare Changed over Time?" Peterson-KFF Health System Tracker, December 15, 2023. healthsystemtracker.org/chart-collection/us-spending-healthcare-changed-time/.

"Provisional Life Expectancy Estimates for 2020." CDC Vital Statistics Rapid Release, 2020. cdc.gov/nchs/data/vsrr/vsrr015-508.pdf.

"Products - Health e Stats - Changes in Life Expectancy at Birth, 2010–2018." Centers for Disease Control and Prevention, January 30, 2020. cdc.gov/nchs/data/hestat/life-expectancy/life-expectancy-2018.htm.

Broaddus, Matt. "Medicaid Expansion Has Saved at Least 19,000 Lives, New Research Finds." Center on Budget and Policy Priorities, November 6, 2019. cbpp.org/research/health/medicaid-expansion-has-saved-at-least-19000-lives-new-research-finds.

Pearl, Robert. "How Health Insurance Became America's Biggest Hustle." Forbes, November 2, 2021. forbes.com/sites/robertpearl/2021/03/01/how-health-insurance-became-americas-biggest-hustle/.

Kelly, Susan. "Nearly Half of Consumers Are in Debt Due to Medical Bills, Survey Finds." Healthcare Dive, October 26, 2022. healthcaredive.com/news/american-consumers-medical-debt-Babylon/634968/.

Bibliography

"Economic Well-Being of U.S. Households in 2022." Federal Reserve Board, 2022. federalreserve.gov/publications/files/2022-report-economic-well-being-us-households-202305.pdf.

Neuman, Tricia, and Eric Lopez. "How Much More than Medicare Do Private Insurers Pay? A Review of the Literature." KFF, May 1, 2020. kff.org/medicare/issue-brief/how-much-more-than-medicare-do-private-insurers-pay-a-review-of-the-literature/.

"Paying for It: How Health Care Costs and Medical Debt Are Making Americans Sicker and Poorer." Commonwealth Fund, October 26, 2023. commonwealthfund.org/publications/surveys/2023/oct/paying-for-it-costs-debt-americans-sicker-poorer-2023-affordability-survey.

"Private Health Plans During 2020 Paid Hospitals 224 Percent of What Medicare Would Pay." RAND Office of Media Relations, 2022. rand.org/news/press/2022/05/17.html.

Brot-Goldberg, Zarek, Samantha Burn, and Timothy Layton. "Rationing Medicine Through Bureaucracy: Authorization Restrictions in Medicare." Becker-Friedman Institute Report, January 2023. bfi.uchicago.edu/wp-content/uploads/2023/01/BFI_WP_2023-08.pdf.

"2022 AMA Prior Authorization (PA) Physician Survey." American Medical Association, 2022. ama-assn.org/system/files/prior-authorization-survey.pdf.

Lubell, Jennifer. "Medicare Physician Pay System Needs a Real Fix-Not More Patches." American Medical Association, January 20, 2023. ama-assn.org/practice-management/medicare-medicaid/medicare-physician-pay-system-needs-real-fix-not-more-patches.

"Medicaid Enrollment and Unwinding Tracker." KFF, March 20, 2024. kff.org/medicaid/issue-brief/medicaid-enrollment-and-unwinding-tracker/.

Berryman, Lauren. "Are Insurers Using Tech to Automate Claims Denials?" Modern Healthcare, 2023. modernhealthcare.com/insurance/unitedhealth-cigna-lawsuits-ai-automation-claims-denials.

Lagasse, Jeff. "UnitedHealth AI Algorithm Allegedly Led to Medicare Advantage Denials, Lawsuit Claims." Healthcare Finance News, 2023. healthcarefinancenews.com/news/unitedhealth-ai-algorithm-allegedly-led-medicare-advantage-denials-lawsuit-claims.

Eisenberg, Richard. "Prior Authorization Rules Are Stressful for Medicare Advantage Customers." Fortune Well, December 16, 2023. fortune.com/well/2023/04/24/changes-coming-to-medicare-advantage-prior-authorization-rules/.

Picchi, Aimee. "Republicans Want to Push Social Security, Medicare Eligibility Age to 70." CBS News, November 2022. cbsnews.com/news/social-security-medicare-republican-proposal-to-boost-eligibility-age-to-70.

Hagey, Keach, and Asa Fitch. "Sam Altman Seeks Trillions of Dollars to Reshape Business of Chips and AI." Wall Street Journal, February 8, 2024. wsj.com/tech/ai/sam-altman-seeks-trillions-of-dollars-to-reshape-business-of-chips-and-ai-89ab3db0.

11.5. ChatGPT's Analysis of 'The Road to AI-Empowered Healthcare'
ChatGPT, 2024. chat.openai.com/.

12. Systemness

"Prioritizing Systemness in Healthcare Provider Organizations." Modern Healthcare Report, 2022. modernhealthcare.com/assets/pdf/CH11452535.PDF.

Stokes, Charles D., and Rod Brace. "Systemness Taps the Power of Interdependence in Healthcare." Frontiers of Health Services Management 37, no. 4 (2021): 17–27. doi.org/10.1097/hap.0000000000000110.

Rubenstein, David A. "Systemness: leading healthcare systems from theory to reality." Frontiers of Health Services Management 37, no. 4 (2021): 28-33.

Tomasik, Jennifer, Brooke Tyson Hynes, and Rosa M. Colon-Kolacko. "Accelerating systemness through shared vision and culture." Management in Healthcare 8, no. 1 (2023): 41-56.

Decker, Christina Freese, and Thomas H. Lee. "Cultivating "Systemness" to Create Personalized, High-Reliability Health Care." NEJM Catalyst 4, no. 3 (2018).

Patricia Salber, MD. "Dr Robert Pearl's 4 Pillars of Healthcare Transformation." The Doctor Weighs In, January 22, 2019. thedoctorweighsin.com/dr-robert-pearls-four-pillars-of-healthcare-transformation/.

Pearl, Robert. "The Middleman Mentality Is Killing American Medicine." Forbes, November 8, 2022. forbes.com/sites/robertpearl/2022/09/26/the-middleman-mentality-is-killing-american-medicine/.

Weaver, Eric. "EP 43 – How the Culture of Medicine Kills Doctors and Patients (Part 1), with Dr. Robert Pearl." The Race to Value Podcast, January 9, 2023. racetovalue.org/how-the-culture-of-medicine-kills-doctors-and-patients-part-1-with-dr-robert-pearl/.

Pearl, Robert. "Breaking the Rules of Healthcare: Paying Your Doctor." Forbes, January 27, 2022. forbes.com/sites/robertpearl/2022/01/25/breaking-the-rules-of-healthcare-paying-your-doctor/.

Haelle, Tara. "Fee-for-Service Still Dominates in United States." Medscape, March 8, 2016. medscape.com/viewarticle/860203.

Shrank, William H., Teresa L. Rogstad, and Natasha Parekh. "Waste in the US Health Care System." JAMA 322, no. 15 (October 15, 2019): 1501. doi.org/10.1001/jama.2019.13978.

Goodson, John D., Arlene S. Bierman, Oliver Fein, et al. "The Future of Capitation the Physician Role in Managing Change in Practice." Journal of General Internal Medicine 16, no. 4 (April 2001): 250–56. doi.org/10.1046/j.1525-1497.2001.016004250.x.

Brown, Christopher. "Health Care Clings to Faxes as U.S. Pushes Electronic Records." Bloomberg Law, November 4, 2021. news.bloomberglaw.com/health-law-and-business/health-care-clings-to-faxes-as-u-s-pushes-electronic-records.

Pearl, Robert. "Why Big Tech Companies Won't Solve Healthcare's Biggest Challenges." Forbes, December 16, 2019. forbes.com/sites/robertpearl/2019/12/16/big-tech/.

Pearl, Robert. "Amazon vs. Apple: Only One Will Rewrite the Rules of Healthcare." Forbes, October 5, 2023. forbes.com/sites/robertpearl/2022/08/29/amazon-vs-apple-only-one-will-rewrite-the-rules-of-healthcare/.

Lawrence, Herman. "Was the Apple Heart Study Virtually Useless?" PCE Homepage, April 12, 2019. practicingclinicians.com/the-exchange/was-the-apple-heart-study-virtually-useless-.

Gonzalez, Robbie. "The New ECG Apple Watch Could Do More Harm than Good." Wired, September 13, 2018. wired.com/story/ecg-apple-watch/.

"Important Safety Information for Apple Vision Pro." Apple Support, 2024. support.apple.com/guide/apple-vision-pro/important-safety-information-c0c84db82a44/visionos.

Pearl, Robert. "Retail Giants vs. Health Systems: Fight Will Come down to 'Systemness.'" Forbes, July 31, 2023. forbes.com/sites/robertpearl/2023/07/24/retail-giants-vs-health-systems-fight-will-come-down-to-systemness/.

13. From Catalog Kings to Healthcare Disruptors

Formichella, Janice. "The Early History of Mail-Order Catalogs." Recollections Blog, February 20, 2023. recollections.biz/blog/the-early-history-of-mail-order-catalogs/.

"The Rise and Fall of Chicago's Mail Order Giants." WTTW Chicago, November 13, 2023. interactive.wttw.com/chicago-stories/rise-and-fall-of-the-mail-order-giants/the-rise-and-fall-of-chicagos-mail-order-giants.

Reiff, Nathan. "10 Biggest Companies in the World." Investopedia, January 31, 2024. investopedia.com/articles/active-trading/111115/why-all-worlds-top-10-companies-are-american.asp.

Reed, Tina. "How Major Retailers Are Trying to Change How America Consumes Healthcare." Axios Vitals, March 8, 2023. axios.com/2023/03/08/how-major-retailers-how-america-health-care.

Bibliography

Pearl, Robert. "Value-Based Healthcare Battle: Kaiser-Geisinger vs. Amazon, CVS, Walmart." Forbes, July 19, 2023. forbes.com/sites/robertpearl/2023/07/17/value-based-healthcare-battle-kaiser-geisinger-vs-amazon-cvs-walmart/.

Pearl, Robert. "Amazon, CVS, Walmart Are Playing Healthcare's Long Game." Forbes, October 12, 2022. forbes.com/sites/robertpearl/2022/10/10/amazon-cvs-walmart-are-playing-healthcares-long-game/.

"Our Take: Amazon Plans to Acquire Primary Care Provider One Medical for $3.9 Billion." Darwin Research Group, July 24, 2022. darwinresearch.com/our-take-amazon-plans-to-acquire-primary-care-provider-one-medical-for-3-9-billion/.

Pifer, Rebecca. "Walmart Health Plans Clinic Expansion in 2024, Pushing into 2 New States." Healthcare Dive, March 2, 2023. healthcaredive.com/news/walmart-health-plans-double-medical-centers-in-2024/643922/.

Minemyer, Paige. "Walmart Enlists UnitedHealth Group for 10-Year Value-Based Care Partnership." Fierce Healthcare, September 7, 2022. fiercehealthcare.com/payers/walmart-enlists-unitedhealth-group-10-year-value-based-care-partnership.

Timsina, Nilutpal. "Walmart to Explore Buying Majority Stake in ChenMed." Nasdaq, September 8, 2023. nasdaq.com/articles/walmart-to-explore-buying-majority-stake-in-chenmed-bloomberg-news.

Richman, Eli. "CVS Closes $69B Acquisition of Aetna in a 'transformative Moment' for the Industry." Fierce Healthcare, November 28, 2018. fiercehealthcare.com/payer/cvs-closes-69-billion-acquisition-aetna.

Terlep, Sharon. "CVS Agrees to Buy Home-Healthcare Company Signify for $8 Billion." Wall Street Journal, September 5, 2022. wsj.com/articles/cvs-announces-deal-to-acquire-home-healthcare-company-signify-11662411855.

Gregg, Aaron. "CVs to Buy Oak Street Health for $10.6 Billion - The Washington Post." The Washington Post, February 8, 2023. washingtonpost.com/business/2023/02/08/cvs-oak-street-deal/.

Reed, Tina. "Walmart Health Eyes Medicare Advantage Business with Planned Expansion." Axios, March 3, 2023. axios.com/2023/03/03/walmart-health-medicare-advantage-business-expansion.

"Top Reasons behind Retail, Medicare Advantage Plan Partnerships." Health Payer Intelligence, September 18, 2023. healthpayerintelligence.com/features/top-reasons-behind-retail-medicare-advantage-plan-partnerships.

Pearl, Robert. "Opinion: How to Get America's Health Care System from Worst to First." The Fulcrum, October 20, 2021. thefulcrum.us/business-democracy/health-care-costs.

Japsen, Bruce. "Walmart and UnitedHealth Group Launch Medicare Advantage Partnership." Forbes, September 9, 2022. forbes.com/sites/brucejapsen/2022/09/07/walmart-and-unitedhealth-group-launch-medicare-advantage-partnership/.

Staff, America Counts. "2020 Census Will Help Policymakers Prepare for the Incoming Wave of Aging Boomers." Census.gov, February 25, 2022. census.gov/library/stories/2019/12/by-2030-all-baby-boomers-will-be-age-65-or-older.html.

Landi, Heather. "AWS Rolls Out Generative AI Service for Healthcare Documentation Software." Fierce Healthcare, July 27, 2023. fiercehealthcare.com/ai-and-machine-learning/aws-rolls-out-generative-ai-service-healthcare-documentation-software.

Blachford, Ashley. "Is Four Times a Charm for Walmart (or, Could Walmart Be a Threat to Urgent Care)?" Journal of Urgent Care Medicine, May 1, 2020. jucm.com/is-four-times-a-charm-for-walmart-or-could-walmart-be-a-threat-to-urgent-care/.

Landi, Heather. "Amazon Care Is Shutting down at the End of 2022. Here's Why." Fierce Healthcare, August 24, 2022. fiercehealthcare.com/health-tech/amazon-care-shutting-down-end-2022-tech-giant-said-virtual-primary-care-business-wasnt.

14. Breaking the Rules

Pearl, Robert. "Breaking the Rules of Healthcare: Selecting the Best Doctors." Forbes, January 12, 2022. forbes.com/sites/robertpearl/2022/01/11/breaking-the-rules-of-healthcare-selecting-the-best-doctors/.

Pearl, Robert. "Breaking the Rules of Healthcare: Restoring the Value of Primary Care." Forbes, March 2, 2022. forbes.com/sites/robertpearl/2022/02/28/breaking-the-rules-of-healthcare-restoring-the-value-of-primary-care/.

Steinwald, Bruce, Paul B. Ginsburg, and Caitlin Brandt. "We Need More Primary Care Physicians: Here's Why and How." Brookings, March 9, 2022. brookings.edu/articles/we-need-more-primary-care-physicians-heres-why-and-how/.

Konitzer, Jacob, and Andrew de la Pena. "The Value of Primary Care from a Payer's Perspective." ECG Management Consultants, 2022. ecgmc.com/insights/blog/1592/the-value-of-primary-care-from-a-payers-perspective.

Kane, Leslie. "Medscape Physician Compensation Report 2023: Your Income vs Your Peers'." Medscape, 2023. medscape.com/slideshow/2023-compensation-overview-6016341.

Pearl, Robert. "Breaking the Rules of Healthcare: The Doctor-Patient Power Dynamic." Forbes, April 14, 2022. forbes.com/sites/robertpearl/2022/04/11/breaking-the-rules-of-healthcare-the-doctor-patient-power-dynamic/.

Pearl, Robert. "Breaking the Rules of Healthcare: Getting the Quality of Care You Pay For." Forbes, April 14, 2022. forbes.com/sites/robertpearl/2022/03/28/breaking-the-rules-of-healthcare-getting-the-quality-of-care-you-pay-for/.

Miller, Jake. "Pay-for-Performance Fails to Perform." Harvard Medical School, November 27, 2017. hms.harvard.edu/news/pay-performance-fails-perform.

Staff, Stanford GSB. "Managed Care: What Went Wrong? Can It Be Fixed?" Stanford Graduate School of Business, November 1, 1999. gsb.stanford.edu/insights/managed-care-what-went-wrong-can-it-be-fixed.

Ikegami, Naoki. "Fee-for-Service Payment – an Evil Practice That Must Be Stamped Out?" International Journal of Health Policy and Management 4, no. 2 (February 6, 2015): 57–59. doi.org/10.15171/ijhpm.2015.26.

Hunter, Kaitlin, David Kendall, and Ladan Ahmadi. "The Case Against Fee-for-Service Health Care." Third Way, September 9, 2021. thirdway.org/report/the-case-against-fee-for-service-health-care.

Lyu, Heather, Tim Xu, Daniel Brotman, Brandan Mayer-Blackwell, et al. "Overtreatment in the United States." PLOS ONE 12, no. 9 (September 6, 2017). doi.org/10.1371/journal.pone.0181970.

Staff, Medical Economics. "Top Challenges of 2022, No. 5: Loss of Trust in Physicians." Medical Economics, January 11, 2022. medicaleconomics.com/view/top-challenges-of-2022-no-5-loss-of-trust-in-physicians.

Pearl, Robert. "Breaking the Rules of Healthcare: Selecting the Best Technology." Forbes, October 5, 2023. forbes.com/sites/robertpearl/2022/02/14/breaking-the-rules-of-healthcare-selecting-the-best-tech/.

Tilburt, Jon C., Matthew K. Wynia, Robert D. Sheeler, et al. "Views of US Physicians about Controlling Health Care Costs." JAMA 310, no. 4 (July 24, 2013): 380. doi.org/10.1001/jama.2013.8278.

Bakalar, Nicholas. "Are Robotic Surgeries Really Better?" The New York Times, August 16, 2021. nytimes.com/2021/08/16/well/live/robotic-surgery-benefits.html.

Pearl, Robert. "Why Telemedicine Is Much More than a Digital Doctor's Office." Forbes, January 31, 2021. forbes.com/sites/robertpearl/2021/02/01/why-telemedicine-is-much-more-than-a-digital-doctors-office/.

Pearl, Robert. "The Anatomy of Healthcare Leadership: A Mind for Technology." LinkedIn, November 14, 2022. linkedin.com/pulse/anatomy-healthcare-leadership-mind-technology-robert-pearl-m-d-/?trk=pulse-article.

"Robotic Surgery Devices Market Size, Growth Rate, Share, and Forecast to 2033." The Business Research Company, 2023. thebusinessresearchcompany.com/report/robotic-surgery-devices-global-market-report.

Xu, Ding, Weigang Lou, Ming Li, Jingwei Xiao, Hongbao Wu, and Jianming Chen. "Current Status of Robot-assisted Surgery in the Clinical Application of Trauma Orthopedics in China: A Systematic Review." Health Science Reports 5, no. 6 (November 2022). doi.org/10.1002/hsr2.930.

Bendix, Jeffrey. "More than 90% of Docs Feeling Burned out: Survey." Medical Economics, February 21, 2024. medicaleconomics.com/view/more-than-90-of-docs-feeling-burned-out-survey.

Mazzolini, Chris. "9 Things Ruining Medicine for Physicians." Medical Economics, November 12, 2020. medicaleconomics.com/view/9-things-ruining-medicine-physicians.

Nelson, Hannah. "Oracle Announces Generative AI EHR Tool for Clinical Documentation." EHR Intelligence, September 18, 2023. ehrintelligence.com/news/oracle-announces-generative-ai-ehr-tool-for-clinical-documentation.

Adams, Katie. "Epic Is Integrating Abridge's Generative AI Tool into Its EHR." MedCity News, August 23, 2023. medcitynews.com/2023/08/epic-ehr-healthcare-generative-ai/.

Jennings, Katie. "Why $4.6 Billion Health Records Giant Epic Is Betting Big on Generative AI." Forbes, March 18, 2024. forbes.com/sites/katiejennings/2024/03/18/why-46-billion-health-records-giant-epic-is-betting-big-on-generative-ai/.

PART FOUR | GENTLY

15. Ethics, Privacy, and Trust

Brockman, Greg, and Ilya Sutskever. "Introducing OpenAI." Introducing OpenAI, 2015. openai.com/blog/introducing-openai.

Kay, Grace. "The History of ChatGPT Creator OpenAI, Which Elon Musk Helped Found before Parting Ways and Criticizing." Business Insider, February 1, 2023. businessinsider.com/history-of-openai-company-chatgpt-elon-musk-founded-2022-12.

Porter, Jon. "ChatGPT Continues to Be One of the Fastest-Growing Services Ever." The Verge, November 6, 2023. theverge.com/2023/11/6/23948386/chatgpt-active-user-count-openai-developer-conference.

Barker, David. "GPTs: Custom Versions of ChatGPT." Hacker News, December 2023. news.ycombinator.com/item?id=38166431.

Metz, Cade. "OpenAI Gives ChatGPT a Better 'Memory.'" The New York Times, February 13, 2024. nytimes.com/2024/02/13/technology/openai-gives-chatgpt-a-better-memory.html.

Khemlani, Anjalee. "GE Healthcare Survey: Ai Faces Skepticism in the Medical Care Business." Yahoo! Finance, 2023. finance.yahoo.com/news/ge-healthcare-survey-ai-faces-skepticism-in-the-medical-care-business-150026030.html.

Dhar, Asif, Bill Fera, and Leslie Korenda. "Can Genai Help Make Health Care Affordable? Consumers Think So." Deloitte United States, November 16, 2023. www2.deloitte.com/us/en/blog/health-care-blog/2023/can-gen-ai-help-make-health-care-affordable-consumers-think-so.html.

Tyson, Alec. "60% of Americans Would Be Uncomfortable with Provider Relying on AI in Their Own Health Care." Pew Research Center Science & Society, February 22, 2023. pewresearch.org/science/2023/02/22/60-of-americans-would-be-uncomfortable-with-provider-relying-on-ai-in-their-own-health-care/.

Mok, Aaron. "CHATGPT Is Getting an Upgrade That Will Make It More up to Date." Business Insider, November 26, 2023. businessinsider.com/open-ai-chatgpt-training-up-to-date-gpt4-turbo-2023-11.

Pearl, Robert. "ChatGPT's Use in Medicine Raises Questions of Security, Privacy, Bias." Forbes, October 4, 2023. forbes.com/sites/robertpearl/2023/04/24/chatgpts-use-in-medicine-raises-questions-of-security-privacy-bias/.

Walsh, Sheri. "Most Americans Uncomfortable with Artificial Intelligence in Healthcare, Survey Says." UPI, February 23, 2023. upi.com/Health_News/2023/02/22/americans-uncomfortable-artificial-intelligence-health-care-survey/4801677114829/.

Metz, Cade. "Chatbots May 'hallucinate' More Often than Many Realize." The New York Times, November 6, 2023. nytimes.com/2023/11/06/technology/chatbots-hallucination-rates.html.

Emsley, Robin. "CHATGPT: These Are Not Hallucinations – They're Fabrications and Falsifications." Nature News, August 19, 2023. nature.com/articles/s41537-023-00379-4.

Ortutay, Barbara, and Matt O'Brien. "ChatGPT-Maker OpenAI Hosts Its First Big Tech Showcase as the AI Startup Faces Growing Competition." AP News, November 6, 2023. apnews.com/article/chatgpt-openai-tech-showcase-da850be425aaa269e2915e9e0b1c726a.

Suderman, Alan. "Poll: 90% of Americans Concerned about Cybersecurity." Manufacturing Business Technology, October 11, 2021. mbtmag.com/cybersecurity/news/21771578/poll-90-of-americans-concerned-about-cybersecurity.

Southwick, Ron. "Data Breaches Continue to Plague Health Care Industry." Medical Economics, February 17, 2023. medicaleconomics.com/view/data-breaches-continue-to-plague-health-care-industry.

Broderick, Tim. "There's No Relief from Healthcare Hackers in 2024." Modern Healthcare, February 22, 2024. modernhealthcare.com/cybersecurity/healthcare-data-breaches-2024.

Burgess, Matt. "The Hacking of ChatGPT Is Just Getting Started." Wired, April 13, 2023. wired.com/story/chatgpt-jailbreak-generative-ai-hacking/.

Burgess, Matt. "ChatGPT Has a Big Privacy Problem." Wired, April 4, 2023. wired.com/story/italy-ban-chatgpt-privacy-gdpr/.

OpenAI. "New Ways to Manage Your Data in ChatGPT." New ways to manage your data in ChatGPT, April 25, 2023. openai.com/blog/new-ways-to-manage-your-data-in-chatgpt.

Alder, Steve. "Is ChatGPT HIPAA Compliant?" The HIPAA Journal, December 15, 2023. hipaajournal.com/is-chatgpt-hipaa-compliant.

Adams, Damon. "Leveraging ChatGPT and Generative AI in Healthcare Analytics." Journal of AHIMA, February 20, 2024. journal.ahima.org/page/leveraging-chatgpt-and-generative-ai-in-healthcare-analytics.

Landi, Heather. "US Patients Believe Generative AI Can Improve Healthcare Access, Affordability, Survey Finds." Fierce Healthcare, November 17, 2023. fiercehealthcare.com/ai-and-machine-learning/us-patients-believe-generative-ai-can-improve-access-affordability.

Obermeyer, Ziad, Brian Powers, Christine Vogeli, and Sendhil Mullainathan. "Dissecting Racial Bias in an Algorithm Used to Manage the Health of Populations." Science 366, no. 6464 (October 25, 2019): 447–53. doi.org/10.1126/science.aax2342.

Dyer, Owen. "US Hospital Algorithm Discriminates against Black Patients, Study Finds." BMJ, October 28, 2019, l6232. doi.org/10.1136/bmj.l6232.

Vartan, Starre. "Racial Bias Found in a Major Health Care Risk Algorithm." Scientific American, February 20, 2024. scientificamerican.com/article/racial-bias-found-in-a-major-health-care-risk-algorithm/.

Vasquez Reyes, Maritza. "The Disproportional Impact of Covid-19 on African Americans." Health and human rights, December 2020. ncbi.nlm.nih.gov/pmc/articles/PMC7762908/.

Johnstone, Thomas, Kometh Thawanyarat, Mallory Rowley, et al. "Racial Disparities in Postoperative Breast Reconstruction Outcomes: A National Analysis." Journal of Racial and Ethnic Health Disparities, April 19, 2023. doi.org/10.1007/s40615-023-01599-1.

Rapaport, Lisa. "Nonwhite Patients Get Less Pain Relief in U.S. Emergency Rooms - Physician's Weekly." Physician's Weekly, July 2, 2019. physiciansweekly.com/nonwhite-patients-get-less/.

"Embracing Generative AI in Health Care." The Lancet Regional Health - Europe 30 (July 2023): 100677. doi.org/10.1016/j.lanepe.2023.100677.

Wachter, Robert M., and Erik Brynjolfsson. "Will Generative Artificial Intelligence Deliver on Its Promise in Health Care?" JAMA 331, no. 1 (January 2, 2024): 65. doi.org/10.1001/jama.2023.25054.

Els, Peter. "How Much Testing Will Prove Automated Cars Are Safe?" Automotive IQ, August 29, 2023. automotive-iq.com/autonomous-drive/articles/how-much-testing-will-prove-automated-cars-are-safe.

Lerman, Rachel, Whitney Shefte, Julia Wall, Talia Trackim, Trisha Thadani, and Faiz Siddiqui. "Tesla Employee in Fiery Crash May Be First 'Full Self-Driving' Fatality." The Washington Post, February 13, 2024. washingtonpost.com/technology/interactive/2024/tesla-full-self-driving-fatal-crash/.

Schwartz, L. M. "US Women's Attitudes to False-Positive Mammography Results and Detection of Ductal Carcinoma in Situ: Cross-Sectional Survey." Western Journal of Medicine 173, no. 5 (November 1, 2020): 307–12. doi.org/10.1136/ewjm.173.5.307.

DeFrank, Jessica T, Barbara K Rimer, et al. "Influence of False-Positive Mammography Results on Subsequent Screening?" Journal of Medical Screening 19, no. 1 (March 2012): 35–41. doi.org/10.1258/jms.2012.011123.

Ho, Thao-Quyen H., Michael C. Bissell, et al. "Cumulative Probability of False-Positive Results after 10 Years of Screening with Digital Breast Tomosynthesis vs Digital Mammography." JAMA Network Open 5, no. 3 (March 25, 2022). doi.org/10.1001/jamanetworkopen.2022.2440.

Satariano, Adam, Cade Metz, and Akos Stiller. "Using A.I. to Detect Breast Cancer That Doctors Miss." The New York Times, March 5, 2023. nytimes.com/2023/03/05/technology/artificial-intelligence-breast-cancer-detection.html.

Kubota, Taylor. "Algorithm Better at Diagnosing Pneumonia than Radiologists." Stanford University News Center, November 15, 2017. med.stanford.edu/news/all-news/2017/11/algorithm-can-diagnose-pneumonia-better-than-radiologists.html.

Kessler, Sarah. "The A.I. Revolution Will Change Work. Nobody Agrees How." The New York Times, June 10, 2023. nytimes.com/2023/06/10/business/ai-jobs-work.html.

Wallace-wells, David. "A.I. Is Being Built by People Who Think It Might Destroy US." The New York Times, March 27, 2023. nytimes.com/2023/03/27/opinion/ai-chatgpt-chatbots.html.

Pearl, Robert. "Sam Altman's Wild 2023 Offers 3 Critical Lessons for Healthcare Leaders." Forbes, December 21, 2023. forbes.com/sites/robertpearl/2023/12/18/sam-altmans-wild-2023-offers-3-critical-lessons-for-healthcare-leaders/.

Tong, Anna, Jeffrey Dastin, and Krystal Hu. "OpenAI Researchers Warned Board of AI Breakthrough Ahead of CEO Firing." Reuters, November 23, 2023. reuters.com/technology/sam-altmans-ouster-openai-was-precipitated-by-letter-board-about-ai-breakthrough-2023-11-22/.

16. Misinformation and Medical Credibility

Johnson, Khari. "ChatGPT Can Help Doctors-and Hurt Patients." Wired, April 24, 2023. wired.com/story/chatgpt-can-help-doctors-and-hurt-patients/.

Weintraub, Karen. "ChatGPT Is Poised to Upend Medical Information. for Better and Worse." USA Today, March 16, 2023. usatoday.com/story/news/health/2023/02/26/chatgpt-medical-care-doctors/11253952002/.

Pearl, Robert. "Google, Facebook, Others Must Do More to Police Online Pseudoscience." Forbes, March 11, 2019. forbes.com/sites/robertpearl/2019/03/11/online-pseudoscience/.

Nagler, Rebekah H., Rachel I. Vogel, Sarah E. Gollust, et al. "Public Perceptions of Conflicting Information Surrounding COVID-19: Results from a Nationally Representative Survey of U.S. Adults." PLOS ONE 15, no. 10 (October 21, 2020). doi.org/10.1371/journal.pone.0240776.

Palosky, Craig. "Covid-19 Misinformation Is Ubiquitous: 78% of the Public Believes or Is Unsure about at Least One False Statement." KFF, August 14, 2023. kff.org/coronavirus-covid-19/press-release/covid-19-misinformation-is-ubiquitous.

Rao, Arya, Michael Pang, John Kim, Meghana Kamineni, et al. "Assessing the Utility of ChatGPT throughout the Entire Clinical Workflow: Development and Usability Study." Journal of Medical Internet Research 25 (August 22, 2023). doi.org/10.2196/48659.

Jeyaraman, Madhan, Swaminathan Ramasubramanian, et al. "ChatGPT in Action: Harnessing Artificial Intelligence Potential and Addressing Ethical Challenges in Medicine, Education, and Scientific Research." World Journal of Methodology 13, no. 4 (September 20, 2023): 170–78. doi.org/10.5662/wjm.v13.i4.170.

Haataja, Meeri. "3 Ways to Tame ChatGPT." Wired, December 15, 2022. wired.com/story/chatgpt-generative-ai-regulation-policy/.

Pearl, Robert. "Healthcare Regulators' Outdated Thinking Will Cost American Lives." Forbes, October 5, 2023. forbes.com/sites/robertpearl/2023/04/10/outdated-thinking-by-healthcare-regulators-will-cost-american-lives/.

Tindera, Michela. "Transcript: Is OpenAI's Business Model Sustainable?" Financial Times, February 28, 2024. ft.com/content/21d26403-61aa-4421-a7cb-d2c9d7c80824.

Baumann, Jeannie. "CHATGPT Offers Potential for Health Outcomes, FDA's Califf Says." Bloomberg Law, February 23, 2023. news.bloomberglaw.com/pharma-and-life-sciences/chat-gpt-offers-potential-for-health-outcomes-fdas-califf-says.

Hurst, Luke. "'Profound Risk to Humanity': Experts Call for Halt to AI Development." euronews, March 30, 2023. euronews.com/next/2023/03/29/profound-risk-to-humanity-elon-musk-and-steve-wozniak-join-calls-to-halt-ai-development.

"Executive Order on the Safe, Secure, and Trustworthy Development and Use of Artificial Intelligence." The White House, October 30, 2023. whitehouse.gov/briefing-room/presidential-actions/2023/10/30/executive-order-on-the-safe-secure-and-trustworthy-development-and-use-of-artificial-intelligence/.

Perna, Gabriel. "How FDA Approval Could Jumpstart AI Use in Medical Devices." Modern Healthcare, 2024. modernhealthcare.com/digital-health/fda-approval-ai-medical-devices.

17. The Human Element

Pearl, Robert. "Op-Med: I Used to Be a Skeptic of AI in Medicine. CHATGPT Changed My Mind." Doximity, July 3, 2023. opmed.doximity.com/articles/i-used-to-be-a-skeptic-of-ai-in-medicine-chatgpt-changed-my-mind.

Pearl, Robert. "Why Doctors Can't Cope with Anguish of Covid-19 Casualties." Forbes, April 19, 2021. forbes.com/sites/robertpearl/2021/04/19/doctors-cant-cope-with-anguish-of-covid-19-casualties/.

Maslach, Christina, and Susan E. Jackson. "The Measurement of Experienced Burnout." Journal of Organizational Behavior 2, no. 2 (April 1981): 99–113. doi.org/10.1002/job.4030020205.

Davis, Katherine. "Physician Burnout Is an Impending Health Care Emergency." Crain's Chicago Business, January 29, 2024. chicagobusiness.com/crains-forum-physician-retention/doctor-burnout-impending-health-care-emergency.

"Transcript: Health Workers Face A Mental Health Crisis." Centers for Disease Control and Prevention, October 24, 2023. cdc.gov/media/releases/2023/t1024-vs-health-worker-mental-health.html.

Pearl, Robert. "Burnout in US Healthcare: New Data, Surprising Insights." Forbes, November 23, 2023. forbes.com/sites/robertpearl/2023/11/22/burnout-in-us-healthcare-new-data-surprising-insights/.

"Overworked and Undervalued: Unmasking Primary Care Physicians' Dissatisfaction in 10 High-Income Countries." Commonwealth Fund, August 16, 2023. commonwealthfund.org/publications/issue-briefs/2023/aug/overworked-undervalued-primary-care-physicians-10-countries.

Ansah, John P., and Chi-Tsun Chiu. "Projecting the Chronic Disease Burden among the Adult Population in the United States Using a Multi-State Population Model." Frontiers in Public Health 10 (January 13, 2023). doi.org/10.3389/fpubh.2022.1082183.

"Non Communicable Diseases." World Health Organization, 2024. who.int/news-room/fact-sheets/detail/noncommunicable-diseases.

"Medication Overload and Older Americans." Lown Institute, January 11, 2023. lowninstitute.org/projects/medication-overload-how-the-drive-to-prescribe-is-harming-older-americans/.

Baicker, Katherine, Sarah L. Taubman, Heidi L. Allen, et al. "The Oregon Experiment — Effects of Medicaid on Clinical Outcomes." New England Journal of Medicine 368, no. 18 (May 2, 2013): 1713–22. doi.org/10.1056/nejmsa1212321.

Perry, Philip A., and Timothy Hotze. "Oregon's Experiment with Prioritizing Public Health Care Services." Journal of Ethics | American Medical Association, April 1, 2011. journalofethics.ama-assn.org/article/oregons-experiment-prioritizing-public-health-care-services/2011-04.

Porter, Justin, Cynthia Boyd, M. Reza Skandari, and Neda Laiteerapong. "Revisiting the Time Needed to Provide Adult Primary Care." Journal of General Internal Medicine 38, no. 1 (July 1, 2022): 147–55. doi.org/10.1007/s11606-022-07707-x.

Terech, Kristina. "Sam Altman Hints at the Future of AI and GPT-5 - and Big Things Are Coming." TechRadar, March 20, 2024. techradar.com/computing/artificial-intelligence/sam-altman-hints-at-the-future-of-ai-and-gpt-5-and-big-things-are-coming.

OpenAI. "Memory and New Controls for CHATGPT." Memory and new controls for ChatGPT, February 13, 2024. openai.com/blog/memory-and-new-controls-for-chatgpt.

Gossage, Bobby. "I Asked ChatGPT to Be My Life Coach. the Results Were Surprisingly ..." Fast Company, July 18, 2023. fastcompany.com/90923620/i-asked-chatgpt-to-be-my-life-coach.

Ross, Casey. "A Research Team Airs the Messy Truth about AI in Medicine - and Gives Hospitals a Guide to Fix It." STAT, July 31, 2023. statnews.com/2023/04/27/hospitals-health-artificial-intelligence-ai/.

PART FIVE | NEXT GEN

18. Technology Alone Is not Enough

"1990: Scuderia Ferrari - History." Ferrari.com. Accessed March 23, 2024. ferrari.com/en-EN/formula1/year-1990.

Somerfield, Matt. "The Troubled Ferrari That Was a Game-Changer for F1." Motorsport.com, December 26, 2023. us.motorsport.com/f1/news/the-troubled-car-that-was-a-game-changer-for-f1/4801237/.

Straw, Edd. "Why the Ferrari 641 Should Have Won a Formula 1 Title in 1990." Autosport, December 29, 2017. autosport.com/f1/news/why-the-ferrari-641-should-have-won-a-formula-1-title-in-1990-4988738/4988738/.

Straw, Edd. "The Full Story behind Alain Prost's Ferrari Sacking." Autosport, October 17, 2013. autosport.com/f1/news/the-full-story-behind-alain-prosts-ferrari-sacking-5102717/5102717/.

Pearson, Dave. "Generative AI: 5 Concerns Voiced by Healthcare Thought Leaders." AI in Healthcare, April 26, 2023. aiin.healthcare/topics/patient-care/digital-transformation/generative-ai-5-concerns-voiced-healthcare-thought-leaders.

Raths, David. "Kaiser Predictive Analytics Tool Reduces Hospital Mortality, Study Finds." Healthcare Innovation, December 7, 2020. hcinnovationgroup.com/analytics-ai/predictive-analytics/article/21164596/kaiser-predictive-analytics-tool-reduces-hospital-mortality-study-finds.

Govindarajan, Vijay, and Ravi Ramamurti. "Is This the Hospital That Will Finally Push the Expensive U.S. Health Care System to Innovate?" Harvard Business Review, June 22, 2018. hbr.org/2018/06/is-this-the-hospital-that-will-finally-push-the-expensive-u-s-health-care-system-to-innovate.

Govindarajan, Vijay, and Ravi Ramamurti. "India's Secret to Low-Cost Health Care." Harvard Business Review, April 7, 2022. hbr.org/2013/10/indias-secret-to-low-cost-health-care.

Pearl, Robert. "U.S. Health Care Needs a Wakeup Call from India: Column." USA Today, January 29, 2017. usatoday.com/story/opinion/2017/01/29/health-care-surgery-india-america-disruption-column/97056938/.

Gawande, Atul. "Cowboys and Pit Crews." The New Yorker, May 26, 2011. newyorker.com/news/news-desk/cowboys-and-pit-crews.

19. Leadership: The Fourth Pillar

Barker, Joel Arthur. Future edge: Discovering the new paradigms of success. New York, NY: Morrow, 1992.

Pearl, Robert. "Who's Responsible for Healthcare's Biggest Problems? 'not Me.'." LinkedIn, April 8, 2021. linkedin.com/pulse/whos-responsible-healthcares-biggest-problems-me-robert-pearl-m-d-/.

Lopes, Lunna, and Alex Montero. "Americans' Challenges with Health Care Costs." KFF, March 1, 2024. kff.org/health-costs/issue-brief/americans-challenges-with-health-care-costs/.

Whang, Oliver. "Physician Burnout Has Reached Distressing Levels, New Research Finds." The New York Times, September 29, 2022. nytimes.com/2022/09/29/health/doctor-burnout-pandemic.html.

Pearl, Robert. "These 3 Healthcare Threats Will Do More Damage than Covid-19." Forbes, August 16, 2022. forbes.com/sites/robertpearl/2022/08/15/these-3-healthcare-threats-will-do-more-damage-than-covid-19/.

Berlin, Gretchen, and Meredith Lapointe. "Assessing the Lingering Impact of Covid-19 on the Nursing Workforce." McKinsey & Company, May 11, 2022. mckinsey.com/industries/healthcare/our-insights/assessing-the-lingering-impact-of-covid-19-on-the-nursing-workforce.

Bailey, Victoria. "32% of Academic Physicians Plan to Leave Workforce, Fueled by Burnout." RevCycleIntelligence, December 18, 2023. revcycleintelligence.com/news/32-of-academic-physicians-plan-to-leave-workforce-fueled-by-burnout.

Sarola, Raymond M., and Jeanne A. Markey. "Private Equity, Health Care, and Profits: It's Time to Protect Patients." STAT, July 31, 2023. statnews.com/2022/03/24/private-equity-health-care-profits-time-to-protect-patients/.

Matthews, Sajith, and Renato Roxas. "Private Equity and Its Effect on Patients: A Window into the Future." International Journal of Health Economics and Management 23, no. 4 (May 23, 2022): 673–84. doi.org/10.1007/s10754-022-09331-y.

Pearl, Robert. "Brain, Heart, Spine: The Anatomy of Healthcare Leadership." Forbes, October 25, 2022. forbes.com/sites/robertpearl/2022/10/24/brain-heart-spine-the-anatomy-of-healthcare-leadership/.

"Top 105 Health Care Unicorns in 2024." Failory, January 22, 2024. failory.com/startups/health-care-unicorns.

Baxter, Amy. "Inflation Eating Away Hospital Margins." Health Exec, July 21, 2022. healthexec.com/topics/healthcare-management/healthcare-economics/inflation-eating-away-hospital-margins.

Pearl, Robert. "3 Surprising Lessons U.S. Medicine Can Learn from around the World." Forbes, February 20, 2024. forbes.com/sites/robertpearl/2024/02/12/3-surprising-lessons-us-medicine-can-learn-from-around-the-world.

Latham, Will. "Herding Cats." MGMA, 2015. mgma.com/articles/herding-cats.

Pearl, Robert. "The Anatomy of Healthcare Leadership: A Mind for Technology." Forbes, October 5, 2023. forbes.com/sites/robertpearl/2022/11/14/the-anatomy-of-healthcare-leadership-a-mind-for-technology/.

Pearl, Robert. "Healthcare Leadership: Following the Money Can Lead to Positive Change." Forbes, December 1, 2022. forbes.com/sites/robertpearl/2022/11/29/healthcare-leadership-following-the-money-can-lead-to-positive-change/.

20. Pole Position

Lansing, Alfred. Endurance: Shackleton's Incredible voyage. New York: Basic Books, a member of the Perseus Books Group, 2014.

Shackleton, Ernest Henry, Fergus Fleming, and Frank Hurley. South: The endurance expedition. London: Penguin Books, 2015.

Morrell, Margot, and Stephanie Capparell. Shackleton's Way: Leadership Lessons from the Great Antarctic Explorer. London: Nicholas Brealey, 2012.

Koehn, Nancy F. "Leadership Lessons from the Shackleton Expedition." The New York Times, December 24, 2011. nytimes.com/2011/12/25/business/leadership-lessons-from-the-shackleton-expedition.html.

Lagace, Martha. "Ernest Shackleton: The Entrepreneur of Survival." Harvard Business School, December 5, 2014. hbs.edu/news/articles/Pages/shackleton-anniversary.aspx.

Pearl, Robert. "Healthcare Leadership: Making Medicine A Team Sport." Forbes, December 13, 2022. forbes.com/sites/robertpearl/2022/12/12/healthcare-leadership-making-medicine-a-team-sport/.

Bibliography **245**

Dean, Bari Faye. "Do You Have the Emotional Intelligence It Takes to Be a Great Hospital Leader? ." Becker's Hospital Review, February 28, 2023. beckershospitalreview.com/hospital-management-administration/do-you-have-the-emotional-intelligence-it-takes-to-be-a-great-hospital-leader.html.

Pearl, Robert. "5 Fatal Flaws of Healthcare Leaders: Inspired by HBO's 'Succession.'" Forbes, June 28, 2023. forbes.com/sites/robertpearl/2023/06/26/5-fatal-flaws-of-healthcare-leaders-inspired-by-hbos-succession/.

Richter, Stacey. "EP412: Leadership of the Art and Science of Medicine, with Robert Pearl, MD." Relentless Health Value Podcast - American Healthcare Entrepreneurs and Execs you might want to know. Talking., September 21, 2023. relentlesshealthvalue.com/episode/ep412-leadership-of-the-art-and-science-of-medicine-with-robert-pearl-md.

"Activation Energy (Article)." Khan Academy. Accessed March 23, 2024. khanacademy.org/science/ap-biology/cellular-energetics/enzyme-structure-and-catalysis/a/activation-energy.

21. Leadership: From A to G

Marquez, Saul. "Direct Primary Care Update." Outcomes Rocket, March 2, 2023. outcomesrocket.health/robertpearl/2019/05/.

Pearl, Robert. "What Healthcare Leaders Should Do to Step up: Part 1." Forbes, January 21, 2016. forbes.com/sites/robertpearl/2016/01/21/what-healthcare-leaders-should-do-to-step-up-part-1/.

Pearl, Robert. "A New Model for Strategic Leadership in Healthcare: The A–G Model." New Leadership in Strategy and Communication, August 24, 2019, 273–97. doi.org/10.1007/978-3-030-19681-3_18.

Neuwirth, Zeev. "Creating a New Healthcare: Episode #145: An Anatomy of Transformative Leadership, with Robert Pearl MD (Former CEO of the Permanente Group)." Apple Podcasts, February 8, 2023. podcasts.apple.com/us/podcast/episode-145-an-anatomy-of-transformative/id1272768725?i=1000598736127.

Cochran, Jack, Gary S. Kaplan, and Robert E. Nesse. "Physician Leadership in Changing Times." Healthcare 2, no. 1 (March 2014): 19–21. doi.org/10.1016/j.hjdsi.2014.01.001.

Pearl, Robert. "Three Ways Physicians Can Become Great Leaders." Physicians Practice, November 15, 2020. physicianspractice.com/view/three-ways-physicians-can-become-great-leaders.

Burgelman, Robert, and Ziv Shafir. "Dr. Robert Pearl and the Permanente Medical Group of Northern California: A Lesson in Strategic Leadership ^ SM333." Harvard Business Review, July 31, 2021. store.hbr.org/product/dr-robert-pearl-and-the-permanente-medical-group-of-northern-california-a-lesson-in-strategic-leadership/SM333.

Centola, Damon, Joshua Becker, Devon Brackbill, and Andrea Baronchelli. "Experimental Evidence for Tipping Points in Social Convention." Science 360, no. 6393 (June 8, 2018): 1116–19. doi.org/10.1126/science.aas8827.

Ahlstrom, Laura. "Ultimatum Game." INOMICS, August 30, 2023. inomics.com/terms/ultimatum-game-1538668#.

"The Critical Role of the Board in Health Care Quality." The Joint Commission , 2023. jcrinc.com/-/media/jcr/jcr-documents/our-priorities/board-education/the-burning-platform.pdf.

Chubbs, Katherine. "Clinical Integration: A Burning Platform." Healthcare Management Forum 27, no. 4 (December 2014): 156–57. doi.org/10.1016/j.hcmf.2014.08.005.

Taleb, Nassim Nicholas. The Black Swan: The impact of the highly improbable. London: Taylor and Francis, 2017.

Alex. "Can ChatGPT Be Both Boon and Bane in Healthcare?" Business Chiefs Insight, September 26, 2023. businesschiefsinsight.com/can-chatgpt-be-both-boon-and-bane-in-healthcare/.

Rege, Alyssa. "Dr. Robert Pearl: My 7 Healthcare Predictions Based on 5 Million People's Data." Becker's Hospital Review, 2019. beckershospitalreview.com/hospital-management-administration/dr-robert-pearl-my-7-healthcare-predictions-based-on-5-million-people-s-data.html.

Pendick, Daniel. "Most Headache-Related Brain Scans Aren't Needed." Harvard Health, March 19, 2014. health.harvard.edu/blog/headache-related-brain-scans-arent-needed-201403197080.

Jang, Ye Eun, Eun Young Cho, Hee Yea Choi, Sun Mi Kim, and Hye Youn Park. "Diagnostic Neuroimaging in Headache Patients: A Systematic Review and Meta-Analysis." Psychiatry Investigation 16, no. 6 (June 25, 2019): 407–17. doi.org/10.30773/pi.2019.04.11.

Sinek, Simon. Leaders eat last: Why some teams pull together and others don't. London: Penguin Business, 2019.

Bowerman, Karen. "Frank Wild in Final Journey out of Shackleton's Shadow." BBC News, December 29, 2011. bbc.com/news/magazine-16165494.

Pearl, Robert. "Five Reasons Why Even the Best of Physicians May Fail as Leaders." LinkedIn, March 9, 2018. linkedin.com/pulse/five-reasons-why-even-best-physicians-may-fail-robert-pearl-m-d-/.

22. Seizing Serendipity

Pearl, Robert. "TEDx: Why Doctors Don't Wash Their Hands." Robert Pearl, MD, October 4, 2022. robertpearlmd.com/tedx-why-doctors-dont-wash-their-hands/.

Ovadia, Philip. "Dr. Robert Pearl: How Artificial Intelligence Will Transform Patient Care #135." Stay Off My Operating Table (YouTube), March 19, 2024. youtube.com/watch?v=uiQjzmUtp8s&t=2s.

Scanlan, Bill. "Washington Journal: Dr. Robert Pearl Discusses Health Care and Covid-19 Pandemic." C-SPAN, 2021. c-span.org/video/?514126-5%2Fdr-robert-pearl-health-care-covid-19-pandemic.

Crane, Donald. "APG Interview with Robert Pearl, MD, Transcript." America's Physician Groups Podcast, July 6, 2021. apg.org/news/pearl-transcript/.

Gaynes, Robert. "The Discovery of Penicillin—New Insights after More than 75 Years of Clinical Use." Emerging Infectious Diseases 23, no. 5 (May 2017): 849–53. doi.org/10.3201/eid2305.161556.

Fey, Paul. "The Mold in Dr. Florey's Coat the Story of the Penicillin Miracle." Journal of Clinical Investigation 115, no. 2 (February 1, 2005): 199–199. doi.org/10.1172/jci24342.

Macfarlane, Gwyn. Alexander Fleming, the man and the myth. Oxford Oxfordshire: Oxford University Press, 1985.

Glasser, O., and M. Boveri. Wilhelm Conrad Röntgen: And the early history of the roentgen rays. Springfield, IL: Charles C. Thomas, 1934.

K., Thomas. The invisible light: 100 years of medical radiology. Oxford: Blackwell Science, 1995.

"German Scientist Discovers X-Rays | November 8, 1895." History.com. Accessed March 23, 2024. history.com/this-day-in-history/german-scientist-discovers-x-rays.

Leonard, Warren. "Serendipity and the Prepared Mind: An Nhlbi Intramural Researcher's Breakthrough Observations." National Heart Lung and Blood Institute, 2013. nhlbi.nih.gov/directors-messages/serendipity-and-the-prepared-mind.

Fry, Alexander Bastidas. "Chance Favors the Prepared Mind." Lindau Nobel Laureate Meetings, July 5, 2012. lindau-nobel.org/chance-favors-the-prepared-mind/.

DeVon, Cheyenne. "On ChatGPT's One-Year Anniversary, It Has More than 1.7 Billion Users-Here's What It May Do Next." CNBC, November 30, 2023. cnbc.com/2023/11/30/chatgpts-one-year-anniversary-how-the-viral-ai-chatbot-has-changed.html.

Pearl, Robert. "How Genetic Insights Can Reshape American Medicine." Forbes, February 29, 2024. forbes.com/sites/robertpearl/2024/02/28/how-genetic-insights-can-reshape-american-medicine/.

Cyrklaff, Marek, Cecilia P. Sanchez, et al. "Hemoglobin S and C Interfere with Actin Remodeling in Plasmodium Falciparum–Infected Erythrocytes." Science 334, no. 6060 (December 2, 2011): 1283–86. doi.org/10.1126/science.1213775.

Barrie, William, Yaoling Yang, et al. "Elevated Genetic Risk for Multiple Sclerosis Emerged in Steppe Pastoralist Populations." Nature 625, no. 7994 (January 10, 2024): 321–28. doi.org/10.1038/s41586-023-06618-z.

Morris, Zoë Slote, Steven Wooding, and Jonathan Grant. "The Answer Is 17 Years, What Is the Question: Understanding Time Lags in Translational Research." Journal of the Royal Society of Medicine 104, no. 12 (December 2011): 510–20. doi.org/10.1258/jrsm.2011.110180.

Gore, Thomas B. "A Forgotten Landmark Medical Study from 1932 by the Committee on the Cost of Medical Care." Baylor University Medical Center Proceedings 26, no. 2 (April 2013): 142–43. doi.org/10.1080/08998280.2013.11928937.

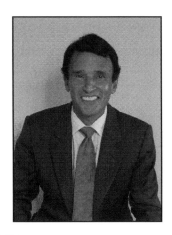

ROBERT PEARL, MD, is a healthcare leader, author, educator, columnist, and podcaster. For 18 years, he served as CEO of The Permanente Medical Group (Kaiser Permanente), where he was responsible for the nationally recognized medical care of more than 5 million KP members on both coasts.

He is a clinical professor of plastic surgery at Stanford University School of Medicine and on the faculty at the Stanford Graduate School of Business, where he teaches courses on healthcare strategy, technology, and leadership. Pearl is board certified in plastic and reconstructive surgery, receiving his medical degree from Yale, followed by a residency in plastic and reconstructive surgery at Stanford University.

He's the author of *Mistreated: Why We Think We're Getting Good Healthcare—And Why We're Usually Wrong*, a Washington Post bestseller, and *Uncaring: How the Culture of Medicine Kills Doctors & Patients*, a Kirkus star recipient. All proceeds from his books, including ChatGPT, MD, go to Doctors Without Borders.

Dr. Pearl is a LinkedIn "Top Voice" in healthcare and host of the popular podcasts *Fixing Healthcare* and *Medicine: The Truth*. He publishes two monthly healthcare newsletters reaching 50,000+ combined subscribers. A frequent keynote speaker, Pearl has presented at The World Healthcare Congress, the Commonwealth Club, TEDx, HLTH, NCQA Quality Talks, the National Primary Care Transformation Summit, American Society of Plastic Surgeons, and international conferences in Brazil, Australia, India, and beyond.

Pearl's insights on generative AI in healthcare have been featured in Associated Press, USA Today, MSN, FOX Business, Forbes, Fast Company, WIRED, Global News, Modern Healthcare, Medscape, Medpage Today, AI in Healthcare, Doximity, Becker's Hospital Review, the Advisory Board, the Journal of AHIMA, and more.

Made in the USA
Las Vegas, NV
06 September 2024

db5247be-cbee-470c-b263-dfbcff0e54a5R01